Veterinary Practice
Management

Veterinary Practice Management

Third Edition

John Bower
BVSc, MRCVS

John Gripper
BSc, MRCVS

Peter Gripper
BVetMed, MRCVS

Dixon Gunn
BVM & S, MRCVS

Blackwell
Science

© 1992, 1997, 2001 by
Blackwell Science Ltd
Editorial Offices:
Osney Mead, Oxford OX2 0EL
25 John Street, London WC1N 2BS
23 Ainslie Place, Edinburgh EH3 6AJ
350 Main Street, Malden
  MA 02148 5018, USA
54 University Street, Carlton
  Victoria 3053, Australia
10, rue Casimir Delavigne
  75006 Paris, France

Other Editorial Offices:

Blackwell Wissenschafts-Verlag GmbH
Kurfürstendamm 57
10707 Berlin, Germany

Blackwell Science KK
MG Kodenmacho Building
7–10 Kodenmacho Nihombashi
Chuo-ku, Tokyo 104, Japan

Iowa State University Press
A Blackwell Science Company
2121 S. State Avenue
Ames, Iowa 50014-8300, USA

First edition published 1990 by
Butterworth Scientific under their Wright
  imprint
Reprinted in 1992 by Blackwell Science Ltd
Second edition published 1997
Reprinted 2000
Third edition 2001

Set in 10 on 12pt Sabon
by DP Photosetting, Aylesbury, Bucks
Printed and bound in Great Britain at
MPG Books Ltd, Bodmin Cornwall

DISTRIBUTORS
  Marston Book Services Ltd
  PO Box 269
  Abingdon
  Oxon OX14 4YN
  (*Orders:* Tel: 01235 465500
            Fax: 01235 465555)

USA and Canada
  Iowa State University Press
  A Blackwell Science Company
  2121 S. State Avenue
  Ames, Iowa 50014-8300
  (*Orders:* Tel: 800-862-6657
            Fax: 515-292-3348
            Web: www.isupress.com
            email: orders@isupress.com)

Australia
  Blackwell Science Pty Ltd
  54 University Street
  Carlton, Victoria 3053
  (*Orders:* Tel: 03 9347 0300
            Fax: 03 9347 5001)

A catalogue record for this title
is available from the British Library

ISBN 0–632–05745-9

Library of Congress
Cataloging-in-Publication Data
is available

For further information on
Blackwell Science, visit our website
www.blackwell-science.com

Contents

Author Biographies

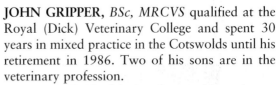

JOHN BOWER, *BVSc, MRCVS* is a senior partner in the Veterinary Hospital Group small animal practice in Plymouth, Devon. He was President of the British Veterinary Association in 1989/90 and also President of the British Small Animal Veterinary Association in 1984/85. He is a founding committee member of the Veterinary Practice Management Association of which he was the president from 1998–2000. In 1990 he was awarded the Melton Award by the BSAVA for meritorious contributions to Small Animal Practice.

He has lectured on practice management topics at the BVA, BSAVA and SPVS congresses, and at all of the SPVS/BVA/ RCVS final year student seminars, as well as at national and international meetings in Denmark, France and South Africa. He regularly contributes articles to the veterinary and lay press, and is the author or joint author of several healthcare books for pet owners. He is a veterinary consultant to Genusxpress, and to Pet Plan Ltd., and a trustee of the BVA:AWF and the Pet Plan Charitable Trust.

JOHN GRIPPER, *BSc, MRCVS* qualified at the Royal (Dick) Veterinary College and spent 30 years in mixed practice in the Cotswolds until his retirement in 1986. Two of his sons are in the veterinary profession.

He now divides his time between consultancy work in the UK, where he is a founder director of Anval Ltd, and working abroad for animal welfare and conservation, where he is a director for the World Society for the Protection of Animals, and Chairman of the Sebakwe Black Rhino Trust.

He is chairman of Rizome Ltd, chief executive of Manor Veterinary Exports and treasurer of VETMIC. He is also a past director of Centaur Services, a past president of SPVS and past treasurer of the RCVS.

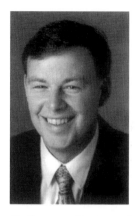

PETER GRIPPER, *BVetMed, MRCVS* is a partner in mixed practice in Somerset and has a particular interest in practice management, business finance and marketing. He is a director of Anval Ltd which offers an advisory service on practice management, finance and practice valuation.

He provides a consultancy service to veterinary practices throughout the country advising on health and safety matters and COSHH, and also produced the Health and Safety website for BSAVA.

He tutored the inaugural Veterinary Practice Management Association course at Berkshire College on Business Management and has given many presentations to veterinary buying groups and pharmaceutical companies as well as at the BVA Pharmacy courses.

He served on the British Cattle Veterinary Association Council (BCVA) for six years and was one of the core organising committee for the XIX World Buiatrics Congress which the BCVA hosted in Edinburgh in 1996.

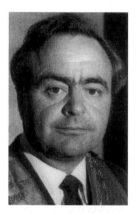

DIXON GUNN, *BVM & S, MRCVS* spent 31 years in a large mixed practice in Cornwall. He retired in 1990 to pursue his interest in practice management.

He was President of the Society of Practising Veterinary Surgeons in 1978/79 and then President of the British Veterinary Association in 1979/80.

He has always been interested in promoting continuing professional development for the profession and his efforts were recognised by his being presented with the C-Vet Award. He is a past chairman of the editorial board of *In Practice*, the *Veterinary Record*'s CPD publication. He has lectured widely on management topics and has numerous publications to his name. Dixon Gunn retired from Centaur Services as both chairman and director in 1997. He is a founder director of Anval, offering management advice to veterinary practices and is still much involved in this work.

Chapter 1
Starting Up In Practice
John Gripper

This chapter sets out a checklist of the basic steps that are needed when you begin your own practice. Starting your own practice may mean taking over an existing practice or 'putting up your plate'.

Further chapters will examine some of the different aspects of practice management in greater depth.

Professional advisers

You will need professional advisers such as an accountant, a solicitor and probably an insurance broker. You may also, from time to time, need to call on other professionals – for example a chartered surveyor, an architect or a financial adviser. A good relationship with your local doctor and dentist will be well worth developing.

The choice of these fellow professionals should be made with care, especially in a small community where it can be embarrassing to have to change at a later date. The most valuable recommendations will come by word of mouth from other self-employed people in the area.

It may be a good idea to choose your professional advisers from firms with partners who are in your own age group as it may be quicker and easier to establish good working relationships.

When choosing an accountant it is important to ensure they have an understanding of veterinary practice accounts and it may be worth selecting your accountant from outside your area in order to find someone with this expertise and background knowledge.

When dealing with other professionals do not be shy of discussing their fee charging systems and working methods before you make your final choice – it can save some unpleasant shocks later.

Bank manager

I no longer regard my bank manager as someone who will give me independent advice – he is employed by his bank and that is where his ultimate loyalty lies. A bank exists to provide you with a commercial service, i.e. the keeping of a bank account and the lending of money. The present day local bank manager has very limited discretion in providing loans and you are best to approach the bank's business adviser and corporate section.

I think that when you first move to a new area you should open a business account with one bank, your private account with another and let your spouse or partner bank with a third. In that way your individual bank accounts will not get muddled and it gives you an opportunity to assess the local bank managers and their levels of customer service. If you happen to come across a good bank manager he or she will probably soon get promotion and move to a new branch. You would be wise to keep an account at the new branch because if you have established mutual confidence he or she could be of great value to you in the future.

Do not be overawed by your bank manager. Be prepared to negotiate loans and terms of repayment in just the same way as you would with a garage salesman when buying a new car. If he or she does not come up to expectations then be prepared to move your account to another bank where the manager will be delighted to welcome you as a new customer.

Insurance

It is essential that you have both employers' and public liability insurance as well as motor insurance, personal permanent health, life insurance, full cover for your surgery buildings and contents, protection for legal costs, and adequate professional indemnity insurance.

Other insurances that you might consider would be for loss of profits, loss of computer records, legal expenses, protection against an in-depth tax investigation, accident and sickness cover, critical illness, private medical treatment, loss of driving licence, loss of credit cards and family income protection.

Contact the different pet insurance companies to compare their terms and services, and decide which policies you wish to display in your waiting room.

Record keeping

You should keep proper records of all your practice's financial transactions, either in ledgers or on computer. These will be needed so that your accountant can prepare the practice annual accounts, and to prepare your VAT returns for presentation each quarter. You should also use these records to monitor your cash flow and compare your financial performance on a monthly basis to your budget forecasts.

In order to manage the practice efficiently you will also need to keep a diary for visits, an appointment book for consultations, a book for telephone messages, a stock control book for drug ordering, a Controlled Drugs Register, a record of X-rays and of laboratory work undertaken at the practice, and finally a record of accidents that occur at the place of work.

In addition you will need a reliable system for maintaining individual medical records of your small animal, equine and farm cases, with a reminder system for booster vaccinations.

When you start a new business you will have to notify your local Customs and Excise Office and register for Value Added Tax if your turnover is expected to be over £52 000 a year (2000/01). All the services and the majority of the goods provided by veterinary surgeons within the UK are liable for VAT at the standard rate.

If your annual turnover is below the minimum level then you do not need to register. This means that you do not charge your clients VAT but you cannot claim back the VAT that you have paid on your inputs such as drugs, equipment, telephone, petrol and professional service. However, you should monitor your turnover carefully on a monthly basis.

When you start a new business it is usually to your advantage to register for VAT so that you can claim back the tax on your initial inputs.

National Insurance and PAYE

The correct National Insurance and Pay As You Earn deductions have to be subtracted from your employees' gross salaries to arrive at the net payment due either monthly or weekly.

At the end of each month (three months for small businesses) you will have to make a return to the Inland Revenue for the National Insurance and income tax deductions that you have made for each of your employees whose wages or salaries have been above the lower earnings limit or PAYE threshold.

The necessary forms, tax tables, payslip booklets and large quantities of explanatory instructions and leaflets can be obtained from your local Inland Revenue office.

You will have to update employees' PAYE code numbers as instructed by the local tax office. At the end of the financial year you must complete all the annual returns for the practice and issue personal certificates of pay, income tax and national insurance contributions (P60) to each employee.

Contracts of employment

As soon as a job has been offered and accepted a contract of employment comes into effect automatically. The terms may simply be those stated at the interview, or they may be set out in a letter offering or confirming the job.

However, all employees whose employment continues for a month or more, are entitled to receive a written statement of particulars of employment. The employer must provide this statement not later than two months after the employee starts work.

A contract, whether oral or in writing is legally binding whereas a written statement of particulars is just a statement 'for information only' whereby the employer tells employees of the more important terms of employment and which he or she believes form part of the contract.

Veterinary assistants should always have a full legal assistant's agreement which will incorporate the contract of employment. Copies of a model assistant's agreement can be obtained from the British Veterinary Association.

Fee structuring

Before you decide on your own practice fee scales it is worth finding out the level of fees which are charged by the neighbouring practices. It is commonplace nowadays for clients to ring round to compare the cost of routine vaccinations and spays.

You do not want to price yourself out of work before you have built up your own reputation, nor do you want to start by undercutting your neighbours as this has a long term effect of lowering standards and quality of service.

Calculate your hourly rate and the appropriate mark up on drugs and you can then prepare a detailed practice fee scale. This can be on display in the reception area or available to show clients on request. In order to assist the prompt payment of fees and avoid bad debts, it is advisable to offer your clients the opportunity to pay by credit card and the necessary arrangements should be made with a bank to instal this facility.

Stationery and practice literature

You will need headed paper, account forms, invoice books or pads, labels for bottles and containers, consent forms, private laboratory report forms, appointment cards, personal professional visiting cards, vaccination booster reminders and debt collection letters.

Many practices now publish their own practice brochures which set out details about the practice, its personnel, its philosophy, appointment times and a map to show its exact location. It is also useful to be able to issue information through practice hand-outs to the clients on post-operative care, neutering, vaccination, and common illnesses such as diarrhoea, vomiting and kennel cough.

Finally do not forget two most important notices for the waiting room and reception area: *No Smoking* and *Please pay cash at the time of treatment.*

Advertising

Now that the Royal College has relaxed its restrictions on advertising there is considerably more scope for the individual practitioner to spend money on advertising, whether it be in local newspapers, local commercial radio or cable television, or through the practice owning and running a racehorse, or participating in British Telecom's *Talking Pages.*

It is vital that your practice name is listed in the *Yellow Pages* telephone directory among the other veterinary surgeons in the area. There is a choice between the standard 'list' format or, for an extra payment, you can have bold type or even a boxed section.

There is some doubt about the cost benefits of taking extra space through boxes in the *Yellow Pages* because if all the practices do it, it then becomes a self-cancelling process. In some areas the local practices have agreed between themselves that none of them will pay for this extra advertising space.

Advertisements can be put in local free newspapers, various local trade directories, parish and church magazines, or posted up at the local library or post office. They can even be put up on the screen of your local cinema.

Inform the RCVS of the change of ownership of the practice so that it can be listed in the next edition of the RCVS *Directory of Veterinary Practices*.

Each practice will have to assess for itself the return and benefit it receives for its expenditure on advertising and the image it wishes to create with the public.

Who to inform

When you start a practice or take over an existing practice go and see the local police to try and establish a good working relationship with them over the procedure for the handling of traffic accidents involving animals. Go and introduce yourself to the local authority dog warden who deals with stray dogs.

Call at your local knacker and hunt kennels to arrange that post-mortems can be carried out on farm carcases. Meet your local butcher or slaughterhouse to discuss arrangements for emergency casualty slaughter of farm animals.

Make arrangements with your local authority for the collection and disposal of clinical waste. The disposal of carcases will also have to be arranged either with the local authority or a private contractor, who may also be able to provide you with a pet cremation service.

Contact the different manufacturing drug companies and encourage their sales representatives to visit and introduce their veterinary products. Make arrangements with a veterinary wholesale company who can provide you with a reliable service and fair discount on your purchases.

Contact the local RSPCA secretary, the PDSA and any other local animal charities such as Blue Cross or Cats Protection League to find out the local arrangements for treating animals whose owners cannot afford to pay a veterinary surgeon's fees. Make enquiries about any local rehoming schemes.

Contact the local dog and cat boarding kennels to find out their vaccination requirements before kennelling or boarding. Try and meet the person who runs the dog training classes. Offer your services as a speaker to farmers' discussion groups, local schools, Rotary Club and Women's Institutes.

Meet your immediate street neighbours to assure them that you will be abiding by the terms of your planning permission and that they will not be disturbed by howling dogs throughout the night, offensive smells or fumes from your incinerator.

Take an active part in your local community by joining Round Table, the Chamber of Trade and local sports clubs. If you are married encourage your spouse to join, for example, the local church groups, PTA at the local school and local charitable or political organisations. This will give you both an opportunity to meet people outside your waiting room and for them to get to know you both.

Join the local BVA or BSAVA division and take an active part in the veterinary professional and social activities in your area. Finally and most important of all, inform your veterinary colleagues in the area that you are starting up in practice or taking over a practice. Better still, arrange to meet them in a casual social setting. You may well find you are able to help each other by borrowing medicines in an emergency or providing each other with cover at night and weekends.

A good personal relationship with your neighbouring veterinary surgeons can avoid many of the misunderstandings that can occur over supersession cases.

Chapter 2
General Tips
John Bower

This chapter is, in many ways, a summary of what is to follow. Points briefly raised here will be covered separately and at length in the book but this chapter is intended to cover some of the principles involved in establishing, building and (importantly) maintaining a successful practice. While most remarks are directly applicable to small animal practice, most principles will apply equally to large and mixed animal practices.

The premises

The practice premises must be noticeable, prominent and in a good state of repair. It must be obvious to the public that the building is, in fact, a veterinary surgery. An effective way of conveying this impression is to display a large, preferably illuminated, surgery sign made of a clean modern material. A logo is a vivid way of promoting the practice, and if the practice has a website, the address could be added to this sign.

Ample and well-signed car parking is essential at, or very near, the practice. Clients do not mind an extra five minutes drive (perhaps to your neighbouring practice) but they do mind spending five minutes looking for a parking space.

It is a good idea to stand outside your premises, from time to time, look at them hard, and ask yourself 'Would I take my animal to this surgery if I had never visited it before?'

The entrance, porch and waiting room should be bright, clean, free of odour, welcoming and interesting. The shy or apprehensive client should not be put off at this stage. Preferably the receptionist or nurse area should be open to, or in the waiting room to make clients feel more at home and encourage conversation.

To be successful veterinary surgeons must be available when the client needs them and to this end it is worth considering very seriously an all-day surgery, preferably by appointment.

The receptionist should be chosen very carefully. She or he is one of the most important members of the practice and must like people as well as animals. She must be trained to greet clients by name as if she knows them and their pet very well – which indeed with time will be the case.

An efficient clinical record system should be established and maintained, and these records, whether on the computer or case history cards, should be available to, and read by, the veterinary surgeon before he or she begins the consultation with the client.

The client and pet should be asked through to the consulting room by name – not 'next please' – so establishing that the practice knows the pet and the case history well. Always refer to the pet as he or she – never 'it' – and get it right.

Consultation

In the consulting room, the veterinary surgeon should greet both owner and pet. The client likes it and it calms the pet and allows for an assessment of temperament. It also establishes familiarity with the pet and/or case.

A thorough clinical examination should be carried out (and be seen to be carried out) at every consultation – this way nothing is missed and your fee is justified. This is especially true when the appointment is for an annual health check and booster vaccinations when many problems which need attention can be detected – teeth, retained testes, ear conditions or parasites for example. If the patient has a microchip it can be checked, and if not this is an opportunity to discuss the wisdom of having one.

An efficient reminder system for booster vaccinations certainly encourages clients to attend. Reminders should be sent out each year; even if clients fail to attend that year it is worth sending reminders again the following year. Indeed the aim should be to achieve about an 80% return on reminders, and experience has shown that this is more likely if owners that do not respond initially receive a reminder after one or two months.

At the end of consultation, a further appointment should be made for another day if you are not certain that the presenting condition will be completely resolved. The client is usually pleased to see the veterinary surgeon being thorough and showing a genuine concern, and the practice receives a further fee from the case. It is a mistake to expect the client to be able to decide whether the case requires further treatment.

The fee should normally be collected after each consultation, preferably at the reception area and not by the veterinary surgeon. This saves paper work, and many clients prefer it. (So does the practice bank manager.)

In the author's practice, the receptionists often offer dog patients a 'treat' (multi-vitamin tablet) on the way out. The dogs like it, the clients like it and it trains the dog to stop on the way out.

So far, little mention has been made of the need to practise a high standard of veterinary medicine and surgery. This is such a fundamental requirement that it is unnecessary to mention it in a book on practice management except to emphasise the need for both veterinary surgeons and veterinary nurses to keep up to date with developing techniques and treatments. Veterinarians should also let clients know in various ways that this is being done.

Having established that good quality medicine and surgery must be seen to be practised, attitudes of staff members to clients and pets are all-important. In general, each pet should be treated as if it were one of the owner's family – it is. Each pet should be treated as if it were the most important patient of the day – to the animal's owner it is; and it should be remembered that even the most routine anaesthetic and operation is a cause of great worry to the client. All surgical cases should be released personally by the veterinary surgeon if possible, or by a veterinary nurse. This is a good opportunity to demonstrate both professional skill and a caring attitude. For example, radiographs and foreign bodies should be shown and, with other relevant details, explained to the client.

Service

Veterinary surgeons must be available when the clients want their services. This may well mean a late evening surgery. And, of course, we should be seen to take our responsibility to provide 24-hour cover seriously and show concern for genuine emergency cases presented at antisocial hours.

We should aim for an honest and open relationship with neighbouring practices. Growth comes more from the increased services and treatments made available to existing clients than from clients who defect from other practices; the latter is usually a two-way process.

Practice staff meetings are useful from time to time. The value to be gained from such meetings when they are properly structured, both in terms of ideas gained and goodwill generated should not be underestimated.

Practice goals – the practice, or mission, statement

I have become convinced that an anglicised version of a mission statement, which in our practice we call the 'practice statement', can be very beneficial. The wording of our practice statement is shown in Fig. 2.1. We have it framed and hung in many sites in all our surgeries: in the waiting rooms, reception areas, office, prep room and staff room. We hope it conveys to clients that we are a caring practice, but more importantly, we intend it to convey to our practice members the approach to clients that we expect of them.

> Our aim is to provide high quality care for our patients
> and their owners at all times

Figure 2.1 The wording of our practice statement.

Media involvement

Media involvement is always worthwhile from a public relations viewpoint. Local papers almost always print articles written by veterinary surgeons on interesting topical subjects and, of course, give credit for it. Local radio stations are often interested in pet health care phone-ins. Where these are not already in operation in an area, it is well worth a telephone call to the radio station to ask if they are interested.

Other involvement in the local community is well worthwhile: dog and cat shows, talks to local groups such as Women's Institutes. Rotary, Round Table and dog breeders' associations provide useful liaison. Open days and client information meetings are also worth considering.

Above all, however, make every client and pet feel 'special' and always know about the case before you enter the room – even if you did not see it personally on the last visit.

It is intended that any actions suggested in this book, should be consistent with advice and restrictions contained in the *Guide to Professional Conduct*, published by the Royal College of Veterinary Surgeons.

Chapter 3
The Practice Premises

John Bower

There is no point being the best veterinary surgeon in the world if your practice premises are difficult to find or if their appearance deters clients from even entering the door. Equally, if the client cannot park the car easily, then they may well drive on to the next veterinary practice where they know they can park. If the premises or lack of parking deter one client a day, this will mean a loss of about £8750 per annum at an average transaction fee of, say, £35.

Therefore, it is important to pay some attention to the premises. Stand outside your practice for half an hour one day and take a critical view of your premises.

Location and site

- Is the practice in or near the population it serves? Obviously a small animal practice will be busier if it is in or near a large population. If not, consider relocating or opening a branch surgery nearer to the population.
- Is the practice easy to reach, for example, on a bus route or linked to the population by fast roads and not in a jumble of one way streets? Is it near a bus stop, a car park, or tube station? Is it near a shopping centre?
- Is the practice easy to see? It should be obvious that the building is a veterinary surgery. If the design of the surgery makes it prominent, it may not be necessary to improve on this. If not, then a repainting programme should be undertaken to ensure the premises are noticeable and also give consideration to large, but tasteful (veterinary surgery) signs.

These three factors can and should be, taken into account in the design and siting of new premises, especially a purpose built hospital or clinic.

The premises

Look at your premises from the outside and ask yourself 'if I were a new client, would I use this practice?'

The premises should be clean and smart and this applies to the car park as well as the building. Would a coat of paint help? Would a new modern entrance door and windows help? Are there any repairs which need to b carried out? In other words, in these days of increasing competition, there may be many relatively small details you can attend to that would make the practice more appealing and more welcoming. Once inside the premises your extremely capable staff will soon convince new clients that they are in the right practice.

Any 'veterinary surgery' or 'veterinary clinic' signs should be clean, fairly large (depending on the practice site), maintenance free and illuminated after dark for ease of location, but not sufficiently bright to upset neighbours. If necessary, night lighting which comes on automatically using a timer or photoelectric cell should be used to enable clients to locate the entrance and walk in ease with their pet from their car.

Car parks

Car parking must be available nearby. Our new hospital on the edge of the city is surrounded by car parking and has become very busy while our city centre branch surgery, which had been there for over 30 years but which was sited on a one way street with very limited parking, gradually became so quiet that we relocated.

The need for good parking facilities at, or very near, your practice cannot be over emphasised. If these are not available, it may well be sensible to consider moving to a different premises nearby where parking is available. It will increase the number of clients using your practice and the number of times they use it. If you make it easy and pleasant for clients to come to you, then it is completely logical that they will indeed use you more often. One has only to consider the success of the large superstores surrounded by car parking spaces on the edge of towns to appreciate how important this is.

If the car park is fairly small, the practice staff should be asked to park elsewhere if possible so that the maximum amount of room is available for clients. Your staff will understand if the reasoning is explained.

So the premises are now noticeable and prominent, smart, freshly painted and clean, with adequate professional signs, direction notices and lighting and the car park is well signposted and obvious. The area round the entrance and the car park is kept clean and swept and free of litter and dog faeces, etc. What else? Well any garden or lawn should be kept tidy and landscaped. Any windows, curtains or blinds visible should be smart and clean.

Other ideas

Continuing with the theme of making it easy for clients to attend your practice, the following ideas should be considered.

A porch

New dog and cat owners these days are often young couples with one or more children. Thus the provision of a porch at the entrance door where a pushchair or pram can be left, especially if it is raining, is a good idea. The practice should also be accessible to the disabled – a ramp instead of steps, and doors that are wide enough to allow wheelchair access to various areas.

Surgery times

These should be listed on a smart, well illuminated plastic board outside the practice. Any branch surgery should also be advertised with its own surgery times on this board. The emergency telephone number (even if the same as the daytime number) should be separately highlighted along with the above notices. Putting a list of the names and qualifications of all the veterinary surgeons in the practice outside the premises is reassuring for the client. Membership of any national association, e.g. British Veterinary Hospitals Association, or achievement of the BSAVA standard should also be displayed outside. Consider also a logo of your own.

Entrance hall

Once through the front door, the client should be able to identify the entrance to the waiting room or reception area. This should be both obvious and welcoming. A series of closed doors facing the client on entering the practice is a great deterrent.

New premises can and should be designed with flow patterns to direct the client automatically into the waiting room. In older premises, it may well be worth considering a glass door and of course, adequate direction notices – smart plastic or wood engraved notices – not sheets of paper or cardboard stuck on the wall. The floor in the porch or entrance hall should be clean and non-slip. The provision of a large doormat will prevent too much water being taken into the waiting room on the feet of clients and their dogs. The first and most important impression should be of a bright, clean, welcoming and odour free premises.

Waiting room and reception area

The waiting room, in common with the rest of the premises, should be bright, clean, cheerful and odour free, with interesting information freely available. The individual style will reflect the practice's personality – whether clean and clinical with modern furniture and magazines, or comfortable and relaxing with plants everywhere. Whatever the style, attention to detail is important. There should not be any old dying plants anymore than there should be old outdated magazines. However, basic underlying essentials for generating and encouraging business are the same regardless of style.

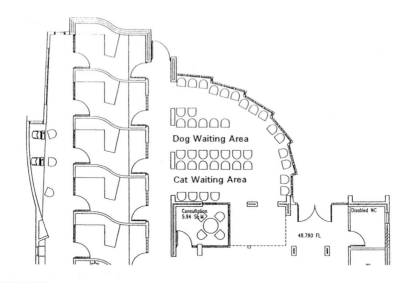

Figure 3.1 Consider separate waiting areas for dogs and cats. *(Courtesy of Form Design Group, Plymouth)*

It helps if the reception area is open to the waiting room so that the client immediately sees the receptionist or nurse on entering the room. A counter top low enough to write cheques but high enough to deter clients placing patients on it is ideal so that the receptionist is in reality almost in the room with the client. This system can be unpopular with the staff to begin with as they feel they need a little privacy, but the clients prefer it. The staff become used to it very quickly. Many direct sales take place across the counter and in addition, discussion will often result in an appointment being booked with the veterinary surgeon.

The waiting room should of course, be warm in winter and cool in summer. If adequate heating is not provided, then this should be corrected. Clients will not wish to stay too long if they are cold.

The walls should be smart and should not be cluttered up with numerous posters stuck on haphazardly. In our own practice, we use a continuous notice board about a metre deep running around the entire room. Cork tiles form the basis of it and this is neatly bordered top and bottom by a varnished pine strip. Using drawing pins, a coordinated display can then be mounted.

It is worth considering the provision of several separate areas on this notice board.

❏ An area for clients to advertise puppies and kittens for sale (remember to date the announcement). The client usually provides and writes out a postcard. No charge is levied for this.

❏ An area which contains labelled photographs of the parts of the practice that the clients usually do not see – operating theatre, X-ray room and wards for instance.

❐ A photo gallery of everyone who works in the practice.

❐ An area for any media coverage of practice or other veterinary activity.

❐ An area for commercial posters covering for instance, vaccination, worming, oestrus suppression, pet health insurance, etc.

❐ An area for details of dog training classes, boarding kennels, etc.

❐ Consider installing the 'stand up newspaper' called *Talking Pets* for clients to read while waiting and holding their pet. This is accompanied by a series of leaflets and is updated frequently to cover seasonal problems, suggestions, etc.

❐ In addition, perhaps a dispenser on the wall to hold your own practice newsletters for clients to take home and one for the BVA:AWF's *You and Your Vet*.

❐ Photographs showing a day in the life of an in-patient, explaining what happens from the time the animal is left for an operation.

❐ An explanation of a serious case with the fees shown, but where pet insurance covered them.

The seating should be comfortable but practical. Plastic individual stacking seats seem to be successful. Any form of bench seating encourages clients to use it for their pets and this can result in problems of defecation and urination.

The floor should be non-slip vinyl with coving at the edges – and of course, should be kept clean. The waiting room must be odour free – and the best way of keeping it odour free is to ask the nurses to look out for and instantly remove any source of odour.

The importance of overall impression conveyed by the client areas of the practice such as the entrance hall and porch, the waiting room and reception area, the consulting room(s) and the exit, cannot be overstressed. Just think of how you feel when visiting a doctor or a dentist and of what impresses you – clean, clinical but welcoming rooms.

The waiting room door should open to a consulting room or a corridor leading to a consulting room or rooms. And why not have a smart notice on this door in the waiting room labelled 'consulting room(s)'. It may also be worth having the facility for an interchangeable sign with the consulting veterinary surgeon's name on – all good communication.

Consulting room

This need not be large but must be well planned. If possible there should be a door for the client to enter and exit but also a separate one for the veterinary surgeon so that if necessary he or she can leave the room at the end of a consultation. It does help to have more than one room for many reasons – admissions by the nurse for surgery, perhaps the room will be very dirty after a consultation, perhaps the owner will wish to stay with a euthanased pet, or a sedated one and the second room means the veterinary surgeon can carry on with his list of consultations.

The room does not need to be large but there must be space for an examination table between the veterinary surgeon and the client (preferably between the two doors).

A hand basin and a small cupboard to contain the routine medicines and injections are all that is needed, plus the computer terminal if one is used. But it is a room in which to do a little bit of selling – of yourself. Have a wall mounted auriscope and ophthalmoscope for the clients to see, perhaps a magnifying wall light, a radiograph viewer, some instruments on a shelf and a chair for the client to use. The examination table should be non-slip and disinfected after every patient (and seen to be – i.e., still wet when the patient comes in).

In any but the smallest practices it is a great advantage to have more than one consulting room either for veterinary consulting or for admissions and discharges, or euthanasias, or just when the main room is temporarily unusable due to the previous consultation. It is also worth considering designating one such room for VN use mainly, as a health counselling, or nurse clinic room.

A one way system for clients – in via the waiting room to reception, then into the consulting room and then out past a different area of reception and out of the practice without reentering the waiting room – prevents overcrowding. This system can be used to encourage payment on the way out by the use of a sign saying '*Please pay here*'. It also gives the distressed owner a trauma-free exit when needed.

Clinical areas

The client of course, rarely sees these important areas of the practice, the clinical areas, which should be equal in standard and finish to the 'public' areas. However, it is very important to inform clients about the operating theatre, X-ray room, ward, laboratory, etc. This can be done in the consulting room by word of mouth, by subtle direction signs strategically placed in the public areas, by photographs in the waiting room and by guided tours involving either groups or individual clients on request. There is nothing more impressive than offering a client a rapid guided tour immediately they show an interest. They know you are very busy and therefore this tour takes only a few minutes or less but they are left with a lasting impression (but the practice has to be one you are proud of!). Clients should be able to see where the dog or cat is to be kennelled during its stay in a boarding kennel and similarly standards in the veterinary practice should be of a level where practitioners are happy to show the client round on request, if veterinary services are to be marketed effectively.

Chapter 4
The Pet Care Centre

John Bower

Most small animal practices, and mixed practices supplying the needs of small animal clients, now find themselves providing some pet care products. These will vary from prescription or therapeutic diets, to life-stage diets, and behavioural correction toys to worming and flea products. As this market has grown, and practices have noted the benefits of retailing such items, so there is a danger of the waiting room resembling a pet shop and leaving the receptionist less time to discuss the clients' needs fully. Nutrition is a good example of this.

The decision as to whether to sell pet care products or not is an individual practice decision – many will think it unprofessional whereas others will feel it is an essential part of the total health care concept in small animal practice. If the practice decides to retail petcare products there are two main approaches.

The waiting room approach

This will be overseen by the receptionist or nurse, and the waiting room will probably house one or more food stands from reputable manufacturers displaying their wares. Alternatively the practice can decide to construct their own display shelving and perhaps amalgamate various makes of food and other health care products into a more coordinated display. Additional display cabinets or stands can be made to look professional and attractive, and a limited level of certain items stocked. There are certainly behavioural correction or prevention tools or toys that should be stocked, from head collars such as the 'Veterinary Leader' or 'Halti' to training discs and occupational chewy toys. It may be sensible to display proprietary prescription or therapeutic diets here to gain clients' interest, although these should not be sold without a veterinarian's recommendation.

Cat carriers, informative books, and an array of shampoos, nutritional supplements and other GSL products can also be displayed. More discreetly, under reception or nurse control, PML products such as flea and worm treatments can be displayed for sale to clients.

If successful, this could grow to take over the waiting room and reception area to the detriment of the professional clinical approach that clients expect. Thus in my opinion, if a practice wishes to pursue the pet health care concept, it may be worth considering a second type of approach – that of developing a pet health care centre as an offshoot from the practice.

The pet health care centre

This progressive idea will not work without that essential ingredient of the total health care approach, the knowledgeable veterinary nurse who has undergone further training as a pet health counsellor or nutrition adviser. If a practice offers a pet care facility, it should offer advice as well. Thus as an effective idea for practice expansion, the development of a pet care centre as part of the practice, either as a new extension or as the conversion of an existing area, preferably as an offshoot from the waiting room, should work.

It should be staffed by a suitably qualified and enthusiastic veterinary nurse who ideally has her own glass walled or open consulting area within it to enable her to discuss, at no charge, clients' and pets' needs. This would be a useful place for the new puppy to have its first outing to the practice, or for the nurse to discuss ways to reduce the patient's weight following a consultation with a veterinary surgeon. There are many such occasions when the veterinarian can refer the client to the nurse after a consultation, so that the vet can deal with the more clinical matters, and therefore become more efficient. It also has the advantage of increasing the status of the nurse and her enthusiasm for the job.

Depending on the size of the room available, the various products should be neatly displayed and able to be handled by the client, overseen by the nurse. The till ideally should be a terminal linked to the practice computer system so that transactions and sales of foods can all be allocated to the patient's records. By siting the pet care centre elsewhere, the waiting and reception areas become calmer and more clinical to the benefit of patients, clients and staff alike.

The natural progression of the idea is that the nurse builds up a following of clients who may consult her for advice. As this advice and help is free, clients are likely to consult her with any worry where they may have been reluctant to consult the vet. They will also call in for food, or for a new flea collar and be encouraged to talk about their pet by the nurse. Worries and queries will be revealed, and the nurse is in an ideal situation to advise a consultation with the veterinary surgeon where needed. Just as importantly, the veterinary nurse is available for advice where in other circumstances the client would have turned to a non-professional such as a pet shop. She should, and will encourage clients to consult her for advice, and this will surely bring more clients in to the surgery. Everyone benefits – the pet gets first class care and nutritional and other products, the owner gets qualified advice and care, and the practice, as well as enhancing its reputation for client care, should become more profitable.

Chapter 5
Client Meetings
John Bower

The concept of staging a clinical meeting for clients is a valuable one in practice promotion. It is an opportunity for the clients to meet the staff of the practice in a relatively informal situation and also for the practice to be seen to be concerned with clients' interests and education.

In outline the practice invites a well known veterinary speaker to talk on a subject of interest to clients, either in the practice or more usually at an outside venue. Some light refreshments are served while the clients mix with the staff and speakers and exchange ideas. At some stage one of the veterinary surgeons should take the opportunity to describe the practice facilities, personnel and their interests so make sure you have some photographic slides of your practice available. A question and answer panel session at the end usually provides a fitting finale to the meeting.

It is important to plan for a clinical meeting at least three months ahead. You will need to consider the following points carefully in order to make your meeting a success.

Topic

Decide on a suitable topic and speaker. Ideas could include canine and feline infectious diseases, behavioural problems and their prevention by puppy socialisation, dentistry, and nutrition.

Budget

The cost of the speaker, venue, refreshments and tickets should be kept within your budget. Sometimes it is possible to interest pharmaceutical companies in sponsorship, although the cost should be justifiable as an item of practice expenditure. Offering a space for a display stand at the meeting may help to encourage such sponsorship.

Fees

Invite a speaker and work out a mutually acceptable date and stick to it. Remember to discuss fee and expenses right from the start. Contact the BSAVA for the current speaker fee rate, and remember to provide travelling expenses and, if necessary, overnight accommodation as well.

In my experience evening meetings are the most popular with clients and 7.30 to 8 PM the most suitable starting time. Ask staff well in advance if they can be available for the meeting.

Venue

You will need to book a suitable venue. We have used a local hotel's meeting room which gives a relaxed setting in a convenient location. It also has the advantage of providing catering facilities. The medical centre of your local hospital may make an even better venue.

Audiovisual aids

Ask the speaker what audiovisual aids are required and ensure the venue can provide them. It is always worth asking if there is back-up equipment if the main set fails, and ensure the room can be darkened. Take an extension lead with you.

Written confirmation

Confirm with the speaker all details – subject, date, venue, time, transport arrangements and expenses – in writing.

Also, confirm with the venue all details in writing. Written confirmation in addition provides you with an accurate record of what you have organised.

Tickets

It is not only interesting to know how many clients will be coming, it is essential for accurate catering, room size and seat numbers. So some form of ticket is needed. The meetings that we have organised so far have been advertised through the practice only to our own clients, although it is now permissible to advertise such a meeting to clients in the press. Bearing in mind that marketing in general is at its most effective when convincing existing clients that the practice can do much more for them and their pets, I really doubt the extra response from broad spectrum advertising is worthwhile – and it certainly antagonises neighbouring colleagues.

We issue invitations to clients in the form of single A4 information sheets about the forthcoming meeting with a tear-off section as a ticket application at the bottom. This should start several weeks before the meeting and of course clients can also be mailed invitations if desired. Obviously clients can bring as many friends as they wish provided the numbers are stated on the form. Simple tickets – overstamped professional cards for instance – are then sent out or handed to the client; and a record kept of how many have been issued.

It may be worth considering raising money for a local charity, BVA Animal Welfare Foundation, or BSAVA Clinical Studies Trust Fund, by charging a small fee for each ticket. This could generate a lot of goodwill and a bit of publicity.

By insisting on tickets you will get a reasonably accurate estimate of the likely attendance, and having asked for tickets clients feel more compelled to attend.

Last minute preparations

A day or two before, confirm numbers with the venue and check all facilities are available. Also confirm with the speaker and check travel and other requirements – including the time that the speaker has to leave afterwards. If the meeting is sponsored, check that the sponsor is aware of all the arrangements.

Remind staff that you would like them to attend and participate.

On the day of the meeting it is advisable for the meeting organiser to arrive at the venue half an hour early to iron out any last minute problems. Hopefully the staff have by now become very enthusiastic about the meeting and will attend to help and mix with the clients. A welcoming glass of wine on arrival will help to break the ice.

The meeting

The following format has proved successful for us at our clinical meetings.

One or more of the veterinary surgeons should sit on a stage or raised dais with the speaker while the audience is introduced to the concept and sponsors thanked. After a short introduction, take the opportunity for self-promotion and give the clients a guided tour of the practice, staff, facilities and perhaps some patients using photographic slides. This should only last 10 to 20 minutes but is greatly appreciated by clients as they are seeing areas of the practice that are normally inaccessible to them and, in many cases, that they were not aware existed.

Then introduce the speaker who, if the subject is carefully chosen, will hold the audience fascinated for up to an hour. This should be followed by a question session on the speaker's topic, bearing in mind his or her departure time.

Whether the speaker has to leave soon or not, I recommend that a panel of all the veterinary surgeons attending from the practice sits at the front for a question and answer session from the audience. This is usually a very popular part of the evening and at our last meeting, I regretfully had to bring the evening to a close at midnight with over half the audience still there.

The clients usually talk about the meeting for days with great enthusiasm. The staff feel they have all pulled together to produce a successful evening and practice morale is raised; not to mention the tales about clients for the next few weeks. The effort put in pays dividends in terms of practice promotion and is another opportunity for demonstrating that the practice is a caring, progressive and enthusiastic team. The secret is in planning well in advance, and keeping in touch with the venue and the speaker. It is a good idea to write and thank the speaker (and the sponsors if applicable) and give some idea of the enthusiasm of the clients for the talk.

Between 100 and 150 clients have attended each meeting we have staged so far and this seems an ideal number. One client was so enthusiastic she wrote a short article on one meeting which was published by *Dog World*.

Chapter 6
Involvement in the Local Community

John Bower

The establishment of the veterinary practice as an important entity in the local community should be the aim of any practice, but especially those with expansion in mind. The practice should aim to have the reputation for being a kind, caring and progressive centre where each case, client and patient is important and where value for money is given.

As discussed in other chapters, practising quality veterinary medicine and surgery goes a long way to establishing this reputation, but there are many ways in which this can be enhanced, and many opportunities to become involved in the local community.

Most areas are now served by local radio stations, either BBC or independent, and these are invariably interested in stories about animals. An approach from time to time by the practice over perhaps an unusual case or species, will often lead to an interview. In addition the local radio stations, wishing to involve the population, frequently broadcast phone-in programmes. Subjects that are always popular are health care and responsible animal ownership, and it is useful to be involved in these if possible. If such a programme does not as yet occur in an area it would be worth contacting the local radio station to suggest it and to offer help. Although always open to suggestions for animal stories, television seems to have a greater requirement for immediacy. It is advisable to establish a policy that the practice will respond immediately to a request for information if at all possible – in between consultations or operations if necessary. Many of these requests lead to an invitation to appear on television, usually on the local 6 PM diary. Clients are always pleased to see their own veterinary surgeon on television especially when he or she is there as an authority on some aspect of animal health or welfare.

Local newspapers

We are all aware how often animal stories and pictures appear in local newspapers where the subject is even more popular than on television or radio. It is also noticeable how often these articles concern RSPCA inspectors, PDSA clients or just the general public. Our profession should become more involved and the guidelines are identical to those for television and radio.

In addition, unsolicited articles, on subjects of topical or local interest, are invariably printed and credit given to the author. I have whiled away many a train journey in this fashion and all articles submitted have been printed.

Press releases on seasonal or topical subjects are an excellent way to generate interest in the local press. The item must be short and snappy, and well laid out so the news desk finds it easy to read. These can be posted but it is preferable to fax or e-mail them to the local papers, addressed to a named contact, if possible. Press releases invariably lead to a short item in the paper, and often a reporter or photographer will visit the practice.

Requests come in from time to time for a veterinary surgeon to give a talk to such groups as Rotary, Round Table, Women's Institute, Young Wives, local consumer groups, etc., and a practice policy should be established on this. I feel it is an excellent opportunity to educate the public on our profession's attitudes, practice facilities and abilities while at the same time convincing them that we are human and approachable. Word spreads and before long requests are forthcoming. The first time you are asked to speak in public is the worst, but it does not take long to realise that talking to a group of 10 to 200 people about life as a veterinary surgeon, or a similar topic really does come naturally especially with the prompt of a few slides of one's practice, or a BVA or BSAVA slide kit.

Specialist talks (for instance to breeders) are more difficult, but in reality these are merely extended consultations on particular topics on which we are all knowledgeable until faced with an audience. The goodwill generated by the talk and during question time afterwards easily compensates for the initial trepidation or even the loss of time off at home.

A long term, and in a way more rewarding involvement in the community, can be achieved with local schools and careers conventions. Here there is an opportunity to advertise the work of the profession and luckily children will sit and listen to stories involving animals longer than any other subject I know. Equipped with a few slides or X-rays, puppy and kitten packs and the BVA's *You and Your Vet*, it is simple to generate a lot of interest and interminable questions, and at the same time preach sound animal welfare – vaccinations or neutering for instance. It is an opportunity to educate the next generation of pet owners. These are the clients of the future and will be likely to remember you and your practice. We also encourage, within reason, visits from schools to our practice.

Dog shows require honorary veterinary surgeons, cat shows require veterinary surgeons to 'vet-in' all the entries. Neither task is onerous, but may involve off-duty time. However, to become honorary veterinary surgeon to the local dog or cat society and to be seen by your clients to be actively involved in these functions gives credit to the practice. It confirms the clients' faith in your practice. Associating the practice with dog training clubs has similar benefits.

These days there seem to be more and more local fetes, many of which now boast a pet show and invite the local veterinary practice to judge the fun classes. These invitations should always be accepted for the goodwill generated, not to mention the enjoyment. If it is impossible for a veterinary surgeon to attend, suggest one or two of your veterinary nurses take on the task – this usually seems to be acceptable to the organisers.

Animal charities

Animal charities are here to stay and fulfil a necessary function. They do not rival veterinary practices in the main and usually need veterinary help. In the eyes of the community, these charities are kind, caring organisations and it follows that veterinary practices that help out with these charities and, therefore, may be recommended by the personnel involved, will also be seen as caring about animal welfare. At local level for example the RSPCA is run by a committee and as veterinary advice is needed, a local veterinary surgeon should be a member of that committee. If the local committee does not yet have a veterinary surgeon in its ranks, an approach may bring an invitation to join.

Opening a new main or branch surgery is a good excuse for holding an open day, but there is no need to restrict the event to such occasions. With well thought out advance publicity an enormous amount of interest can be generated among clients for an open day when they will have the rare opportunity to see around the whole practice and talk at leisure to the staff. Of necessity these events will normally be on Sundays or during an evening, but provided the enthusiasm is there and enough notice given, the staff will usually be pleased to be involved. The occasion is enhanced by a little wine or tea and soft drinks and the facilities of the practice can be demonstrated at leisure.

It is possible to interest pharmaceutical or pet insurance companies in sponsorship of such events and there is normally client interest if representatives of such companies are invited to attend.

Evening events are also very popular – if the ones we have tried so far are representative. The format suggested is to invite a well known veterinary speaker to talk to clients on a topic that is of interest to them and to advertise it to clients for weeks in advance. Topics such as infectious diseases in a kennel situation (cats or dogs), or behavioural problems seem to attract large audiences, so a suitable hotel venue is recommended. We have had attendances of over 100 clients at our meetings and I have heard of still larger ones.

The attitude of the practice to wildlife is important and a policy should be established and adhered to by all staff. When presented to us by a client, an ill or injured wild creature requires the same care and attention as our normal patients. It needs our help and must been seen to receive it. If euthanasia is in its best interest, then we must say so, or if aftercare is feasible and will be accepted by the patient, then we must treat. And as no one owns the animal, we should not look around for someone to foot the bill. The client will have put effort into bringing the animal to us, the practice will normally have access to clients who are prepared to provide postoperative care for wildlife, and so we, in turn, should be prepared to give our time and skill at no charge to anyone.

I am convinced that this caring attitude to our fellow wild creatures on this earth does not go unnoticed by our clients and raises the status of our practices in the community.

Chapter 7

The Receptionist and the Nurse

John Bower

The receptionist

The receptionist is one of the most important people within the practice from the practice development point of view. She or he has the most contact with clients both on the telephone and in the practice itself. Thus, she has the potential for winning over clients or losing them – purely by her attitude to them.

The potential value of the initial telephone contact with the practice should not be underestimated. How many times each day, for instance, do clients telephone to ask the cost of a procedure such as a routine spay operation, or puppy vaccination? Perhaps once, perhaps ten times each day. If the receptionist quickly but politely tells the client the cost and replaces the receiver, how many potential clients are lost on the grounds of cost alone to other practices? If the receptionist, because she wants the client to come to 'her' practice, expresses an interest and extends the conversation, the client is much more likely to use your practice where the patient will apparently be treated as an individual.

It is easy to steer that initial conversation: 'Oh, you have a new puppy/ kitten. Lovely, what breed? Oh, yes, we had one of those in this morning. Are you finding him easy to train? You haven't let him walk on the ground outside your garden yet have you?' etc. Always refer to the pet as he or she – and get it right. Suddenly someone cares about the puppy and the client is much more likely to come to the practice. Usually once there with a new young patient, they will attend for the rest of the patient's life.

The same first impression or initial response is equally important when clients call into the waiting room or reception area. The receptionist(s) must be smartly dressed and if not VNs, should be recognisable as receptionists. A uniform is a good idea, and this can vary from the practice sweat shirt with logo and smart trousers or dress, to a more formal uniform. We prefer the receptionists to choose their own outfits with the sole proviso that they should be smart and coordinated with a name badge or name embroidered on to them.

The receptionist's attitude and greeting to the clients as they arrive is all important. With regular clients, the receptionist should greet them as old friends. We all like to be made to feel welcome wherever we go and our clients are no exception: 'Good morning, Mrs Payne. How is Sheba?' is far better than 'What is your name, please?' With increasing use of appointments and computerisation, there is no reason why the receptionist should not be expecting particular clients to arrive, and should be able to call them up on the screen, or on the day's appointment list very quickly, enabling a knowledgeable greeting and conversation. So it is important to try and have permanent staff in this position and to encourage them to learn to recognise the clients (or at least the patient) and to use their names. And if, for instance, there is a delay in the appointment system or a wait ahead of the client, the receptionist should, at that stage, apologise and explain the delay and the reason for it, and then keep the waiting clients informed and involved.

In the case of new clients, it is important to make them welcome and to feel comfortable in this, their first visit to the practice. It is also important to register them fully and correctly, and a 'new client registration form' that they fill out then or take home to fill out, is a great help. Essential details that are often forgotten will include the names and species of all their pets, not just the one presented that day, pet insurance details, known allergies and old illnesses etc. A good receptionist will explain a little about the practice, enquire how they heard of us, and send them away after the consultation with a 'new client pack' consisting of useful and friendly information about the practice. We always allocate a double appointment for any new client to allow them to settle in and get to know us a bit better.

The approach to clients arriving unexpectedly to make inquiries, or expecting their pet to be given a vaccination there and then is equally if not more important. The receptionist, however busy, must acknowledge their arrival, even if it is just by a smile or nod, and should indicate that she will attend to them just as soon as she has finished dealing with the case in hand. And then she must give the client some time. It is all too easy to make the client feel unwelcome, or that they are being a nuisance when, in fact, the client had no idea how the practice was run. Far better to fit the client in, allow them to see the veterinary surgeon if at all possible, and then train them to the practice system for the next visit.

Thus for practice expansion and client satisfaction, it is essential to have a reliable, enthusiastic receptionist – someone who likes and communicates well with people. If the receptionist likes animals as well, that is a bonus. A pleasant, chatty, outgoing but sympathetic personality is a prerequisite for a receptionist. If one client a day is lost through lack of attention then at say £35 the practice may lose £8,750 per year, as well as the recommendations that may have come from that client over the years. Bad news spreads quicker than good news. A practice can be very fortunate in happening on a good communicative receptionist with just the right attitude and approach, but this should not be taken for granted, and lack of people skills should be tolerated at the practice's peril. Interpersonal skills training is available and should be provided for receptionists as well as for any practice member who comes into contact with the public and would benefit from the training.

The receptionist's (or anyone else's) attitude to collecting money is important. Clients should be encouraged to pay on the way out of the surgery and the receptionist should become adept at politely collecting the fee. She should not be defensive over fees, they are just a fact, but she should be able to itemise and discuss them to ensure the clients understand how the fee is calculated. She may receive many comments about the fees, as do other retail outlets, but her answer should be the same as we receive elsewhere as consumers – 'Yes, isn't everything expensive these days, but thank goodness we were able to help Sheba', etc. A good friend of mine recently took his receptionist to the local supermarket with him to buy items for the practice, then asked firstly if the girl at the check-out could send him the bill as he had forgotten his money, then asked if he could take the items and call back with the money – all to no avail of course – and by then had a cringing embarrassed receptionist who has still not forgiven him! All to illustrate how she should behave when clients put her in the same situation.

In addition, a good receptionist will ask each and every client if the veterinarian wishes to see the patient again and fix another appointment if possible, or at least write the date of suggested return on an appointment card for the client. This is a good way to help expand the practice.

We all have clients who fail to keep their appointments – some just forget, some feel it may not be necessary as the pet has improved, some are wavering because of the fee. A receptionist should always be encouraged to telephone these clients shortly after the missed appointment in a concerned fashion to inquire how 'Sheba' is, mention the missed appointment as the veterinarian was concerned about Sheba, and offer to make another one.

The nurse

It is important to give the nurses status within the practice whether a student veterinary nurse (SVN) or qualified veterinary nurse (VN). A feature on the waiting room notice board, or the practice video, about the practice being a training centre, or about the VN career spreads the word and is of interest to the clients. Emphasis on individual clinical patient care is increased if the nurses are in uniform and wearing a name badge. It gives them an identity. The nurses should take pride in their work and appearance, and have an obvious caring attitude to the patients.

All of the comments concerning receptionists will apply to nurses in practices where the nurses fulfil the receptionist's role. Surely at some time in most practices, even if only dealing with after hours problems, nurses come into contact with clients in person or on the telephone, so it is equally important that these clinically excellent people either have, or are trained to have interpersonal skills too. The love of animals rather than people is no reason to employ an interviewee; both are necessary for this vital role.

Within the practice there are certain specific situations where the nurse has contact with people and clinical skills can be used to advantage. These include the following.

❐ Inquiries over the telephone or in the waiting room as to the health of in-patient pets – from routine neuterings to complicated lifesaving procedures.

❐ Requests for help in urgent cases during antisocial hours – in practices where the resident nurses answer the telephones at nights and weekends.

❐ In the ward when owners visit their pets.

❐ At the time of admission or release of a surgical case or medical in-patient.

❐ On the way out from the consultation, the nurse may hand over and discuss medication with the client.

❐ On any occasion when the nurse will collect a patient from his home for treatment.

❐ As a pet health counsellor, nutrition adviser or other similar role within the practice (see Chapter 8).

On all these occasions the most important impression given by the nurse must be that at that moment, that particular patient is the most important in the world. This is especially important when admitting or releasing a patient for a surgical operation, however minor the procedure. The average client is very worried and concerned about general anaesthesia and even a routine spay operation arouses great concern in most clients. If the nurse is gentle, reassuring and caring and obviously treating the pet as an individual and special case in the client's eyes, that client will leave the premises much happier.

The nurse should be encouraged to use the pet's name when issuing postoperative instructions such as 'do not give Sheba any food tonight' and not 'we advise you not to feed dogs after this operation'. Always personalise it. We have found that issuing written postoperative instructions ensures that the owner remembers all the advice and the best time to issue them is when the animal is admitted for the procedure.

Clinical training of veterinary nurses

Many practices train student veterinary nurses and have in the past been disappointed with the low pass rates achieved in the RCVS veterinary nursing examinations. It was difficult to know how much of the blame for this lay with a practice's training approach, the students, or the system itself. The recent introduction of the new VN S/NVQ, with its increased requirements in terms of time and other resources, although needed, initially seemed unnecessarily complicated with a great deal more paperwork involved than with the 'old' scheme which ceased. This means that a practice must register as an Approved Training and Assessment Centre (ATAC) (a title which may change in spring of 2001) and enrol future students on the VN S/NVQ scheme.

The practice staff themselves require training for the supervision of the students' in-house training, and the students can opt for block release college education for their formal lectures, alternating with hospital based practical training, or day release or distance learning. Initially the practice needs an enthusiast, perhaps a well qualified head nurse, to get started. A talk to the whole practice to explain what is involved is useful as even the terminology is fairly obscure to those not using it every day (see glossary at the end of this chapter). Individuals within the team who can take on the responsibility of supervising the students and the running of the scheme need to be identified. These are the so-called *internal verifiers, internal assessors* and *evidence gatherers*.

It is advisable for every practice embarking on NVQ training to appoint an appropriate nurse or vet to steer and coordinate the scheme, as without such a leader there may be confusion, demoralisation and great inefficiency. This person needs access to the correct information, contacts, and above all the allocated time to get things moving in the right direction.

Internal assessors

These are needed to work directly with the students, assessing their practical work and portfolio log sheets. The portfolio is an extremely important aspect of the student's training and assessment. A student nurse cannot qualify without having passed both their Part 1 and Part 2 examinations, but also having submitted a satisfactory portfolio for both Level 2 and Level 3. The portfolio is much more detailed than the old practical 'green' books. To complete their portfolios, the students are required to write up case log sheets across a wide range of circumstances that demonstrate they have all of the nursing skills required of professional veterinary nurses.

In practice with several student nurses training at any one time, each assessor is allocated a small number of student VNs to work with. Their responsibilities include drawing up their allocated students' action plans, undertaking practical assessments, signing off case logs and regularly reviewing portfolio work to date. The nominated assessor checks the students' work and also attends periodic NVQ team meetings to report on their students' progress to date. Practices are required to devote a minimum of three hours per week to each student on an individual basis and try when possible to allocate time for this in advance on the work rotas. This three hour period each week includes assessment planning, practical observation of the students, questioning and signing off of case logs, reviews of portfolio work to date, and private tutorials. The idea of being able to do this on a regular basis seems at first an impossibility, but with careful planning and efficient working it can be done, and the time spent by assessors with students on a one-to-one basis is extremely valuable and much appreciated.

Evidence gatherers

These are generally other veterinary surgeons or veterinary nurses who observe the students undertaking particular tasks and sign witness statements to specify the involvement and quality of their performance. No specific training is required for this, but students need to make the person aware that they will be asked to sign a witness statement so that they pay full attention to their involvement.

Internal verifiers

Very careful thought must be given to the selection of internal verifiers, who should be either qualified veterinary surgeons or qualified and listed VNs. Training and qualification is required for this role, whose responsibilities are to support the internal assessors, but also ensure the quality assurance of assessments within their centre. Periodically (approximately once every three months), the internal verifiers will observe student assessments and examine the portfolio work produced to ensure that each assessor is adhering to the national standards and that there is consistency between different students, assessors, and elements of the standards.

An internal verifier should be someone who is keen to be involved with the scheme, but also possess the necessary authority to fulfil this role and liaise with the awarding body.

The internal verifier and internal assessor cannot be the same person unless a second internal verifier is appointed. This is because an internal verifier cannot verify their own assessments. Therefore, what often happens is that a nurse will work towards D32/D33 to train as an assessor, with another nurse or vet (perhaps even the principal) working towards D34 to ensure there is no conflict in their roles. Veterinary nurses seem best placed to act as assessors as they work with the students every day, whereas the veterinary surgeons are more suited to the verification role. There are changes in the pipeline which will mean that it will not be necessary to have an internal verifier in every practice, as groups may be served by one individual supplied, for example, by a local training college.

NVQ team meetings

These meetings are best held monthly and attended by the internal verifiers, the internal assessors and the practice manager or partner. An agenda is circulated in advance and full minutes of the meetings are kept. These should be filed confidentially, and are not only available for reference but can also be examined by the external verifier during a visit to the ATAC.

Records

The records relating to the training of student veterinary nurses are filed away in a locked cabinet in order to maintain confidentiality. These records include:

- sickness and holiday records
- assessment planning forms
- assessment reports
- diary documenting informal review conversations
- formal review reports
- internal verification reports
- minutes of meetings
- copies of RCVS newsletters and bulletins
- copies of internal memoranda relating to the NVQ
- copies of correspondence with the RCVS and BVNA
- copies of the CVs and TDLB certificates of the all assessors and verifiers.

These records are available to be inspected by the awarding or accrediting bodies.

Costs

In our practice we received a 45% refund from our local TEC (Training and Enterprise Council) for the fees paid to train towards D32/D33 and D34. (The total cost to the practice has been in the region of £450 to train four assessors and two internal verifiers). There is, perhaps, more cost in terms of time which has included 30–40 hours of study and assessing for each internal assessor and verifier and also the ongoing time involved with planning and carrying out assessments which we are managing to keep to roughly three hours per week, per student.

Benefits for the students

- Students play a much greater role with each of the cases in which they are involved. They are more inquisitive and ask far more well thought-out questions.
- The scheme encourages a practical, case-orientated approach and there is detailed guidance in the curriculum available for both the student and others involved to see exactly what knowledge and practical competence is required of VNs.
- There is a detailed syllabus which helps both students and practice in knowing exactly what they need to know and in what depth.
- The students are required to show evidence, knowledge and experience gained in their case logs. An increased understanding as well as curiosity as to why things are done in a particular way helps maintain interest in the job, and by feeling more involved they also become more enthusiastic and confident.
- All these factors turn them into better nurses, our pass rate has significantly improved, and it is hoped the drop out rate in the profession through work dissatisfaction may also reduce.

Benefits for the practice

❑ The framework of the NVQ helps to set targets and timetables for training, and introduces a positive culture of learning into the practice.

❑ Student nurses are being better trained and rapidly become useful and enthusiastic members of the practice team. They realise a lot is being put into their education, and give something back in return.

❑ Nurses on duty at night are often to be found, during a quiet spell, working on their portfolios or leafing feverishly through practice library books instead of watching TV.

❑ In our large practice, this summer, we have seen a 100% pass rate for all of our students who entered examinations and submitted portfolios.

❑ Training and functioning as an assessor can give new interest and challenges to qualified VNs and a sense of satisfaction through contributing to others' education.

❑ The practice benefits from the team approach which is encouraged by the scheme.

Summary

Student nurses who recognise that the practice staff are investing in their education and training will be far happier, motivated and more likely to stay with the practice or the profession. Veterinary nursing is a practical job which mixes science and art in a similar way as veterinary surgery. The new scheme takes a holistic approach to working with animals and people, and there is plenty of provision for both client and animal care in a practical setting. If the veterinary profession works with this scheme we will reap the rewards of better trained, motivated nurses. I would encourage all those worried about coping with it to battle on as the benefits will be well worthwhile.

Glossary

Accrediting bodies: The Qualifications and Curriculum Authority and the Scottish Qualifications Authority who have given accreditation to the RCVS to be the awarding body for the VN S/NVQ. The QCA and SQA carry out national regulation of NVQs in England and Scotland respectively.

ATAC: Approved Training and Assessment Centre – currently the title of veterinary practices which have been approved to train SVNs.

Awarding body: The RCVS who award the VN S/NVQ. In this capacity, the RCVS are accountable to QCA and SQA for maintaining the overall quality of the award.

Evidence gatherers: These are qualified veterinary surgeons or qualified and listed VNs who do not hold D32/D33, nor are working towards it. They are however, in a position to be able to observe a student's performance and produce a witness statement.

External verifiers: Appointed by the RCVS, these are qualified veterinary surgeons or qualified and listed VNs with a minimum of five years postgraduate experience. Their role is to advise and support ATACs, promote best practice and monitor the quality assurance of assessment activities within ATACs.

Internal assessors: These must be either qualified veterinary surgeons or qualified and listed VNs based within the ATAC who are responsible for assessing a student's performance, making a judgement, providing feedback and signing off the portfolio case log sheets when competent.

Internal verifiers: These must be either a qualified veterinary surgeon or qualified and listed VN whose main role is to support the assessors and maintain the quality and consistency of assessments undertaken within the centre.

Occupational standards: These state details of what the student should be competently capable of performing and the underpinning knowledge they need.

TDLB (Training and Development Lead Body) Units:

- ❏ D32/D33: 'Assess Candidate Performance' and 'Assess Candidate Performance Using Differing Sources of Evidence'. Internal assessors must either be working towards or must have achieved this award.
- ❏ D34: 'Internally verify the assessment process'. Internal verifiers must either be working towards or must have achieved this award.
- ❏ D35: 'Externally Verify the Assessment Process'. External verifiers must either be working towards or must have achieved this award.

Where to get more information

Contact your Regional RCVS external verifier. If you don't have their details, then the VN Dept. at the RCVS should be able to assist you (telephone 020 7222 2001).

The RCVS Training Centre Handbook (available from the RCVS) should be available in each ATAC and contains guidance notes relating to the scheme and the roles and responsibilities of all those involved, but also includes the Occupational Standards.

Chapter 8
Veterinary Nurse Clinics
John Bower

Within most small animal practices these days there is a potential for developing either 'nurse clinics', or merely greater nurse involvement with the client base. As a profession we are now more aware of the benefits of earlier socialisation, better nutrition, a closer eye on that important first six months or so of development, and care of the ageing pet. Much of this can be advice given by an experienced veterinary nurse either to groups of pet owners or individually as needed within the practice.

There is no doubt that the qualified veterinary nurse is a dedicated caring and ambitious practice member. Advancement and responsibility is important to them, and many are taking diplomas, nutritional or pet health care courses. This knowledge and enthusiasm must be put to good use in the practice; the nurse usually welcomes the chance to share this knowledge with pet owners. In many circumstances this takes the pressure off the vets and creates extra opportunities for the practice. The benefits to the VN are those of increased responsibility, career progression and job satisfaction. Some of the ways in which the practice can harness this energy and enthusiasm are set out below.

Practices are quite rightly beginning to regard the nurse as a source of income as well as being a member of the support team for the veterinary surgeons, and will make a charge for the nurse's time in some of the services or clinics described. Others will run the clinics with no charge for the nurse's time as a service to clients that may have sales attached to the clinics, or happy in the knowledge that this free service bonds the clients to the practice. Whether a charge is made or not, the nurse clinic is a valuable addition to a practice's repertoire.

Pre-vaccination puppy and kitten consultations

Owners of new puppies and kittens often contact the practice immediately on purchasing the new pet. Frequently the advice is to let the pet settle in for a week or two at, say, six weeks old, and then attend the vaccination course. This is a time of wonderment for most families and the first week or two is spent fact finding. At this stage a (free) health check and advice session with a VN in the practice will fulfil the client's needs, reassure them that the pet is healthy, and ensure that the best possible advice is obtained on items such as worming, nutrition, pet insurance and socialisation. The new pet owner just has to talk to someone about all this, and to enthuse about their pet, and if their veterinary practice is not interested at this stage, they will resort to other outlets. Surely we have all been presented with pups and kittens wrongly wormed, treated with inappropriate flea treatments purchased from pet shops, and on poor diets, where uninformed advice has been obtained at this stage elsewhere.

This consultation, in a quiet room at a quiet time of the day, shows the practice's genuine interest in this new family member, and usually ends with an appointment for the first vaccination. If the practice stocks food and toys, this is an ideal opportunity to inform the client and ensure the pet has the best possible start.

Puppy classes

Although becoming far more popular and widespread, puppy classes and their value to the pet, owner and practice are still probably underestimated by most practices. There is now no doubt that the properly socialised puppy is a much more balanced individual, a joy to own, and a welcome member of the community. It is imperative to socialise and habituate them before 14 weeks of age, so the classes are usually started a week after the first vaccination.

We hold classes in a branch surgery, on a weekly basis for four weeks, one hour a week during a morning, and the puppy can join at any stage of the course – it is a rolling four weeks which is very structured. An alternative is to hold classes or parties in the evenings but there are implications for staff overtime.

After four weeks, the advantages are obvious. The puppies can't wait to get back to see their friends at the practice, they lose any fear of the veterinary surgery, they continue to learn communication skills with other dogs and other people, and at the same time the owners are learning about diet, worming, training, behaviour, pet insurance and all the other things they have forgotten in the years since they last had a puppy. The practice gains because unfazed patients are easier to treat, the clients are bonded to the practice, and because of the sales of food, Identichip, and other products to these clients – which of course may continue.

Certainly when they reach maturity it is noticeable how well behaved these same dogs are when they return for their first annual booster vaccination. They also seem relaxed and content at being back in the surgery.

Adolescent health checks

These are popular with both the owner and practice alike and are usually carried out at five and a half to six months of age, just as the permanent teeth are almost fully erupted. In our practice a vet will carry this out, with an appropriate examination fee charged, but many practices delegate this task to a VN. We send a reminder for this, flagged on the computer at the time of the second consultation, and with the reminder is a health sheet detailing what we will do and the topics we will cover. The client is asked to bring this form with them at the time of the health check. A full clinical examination is carried out by the vet, or a health check by the nurse, and the opportunity is used to discuss development and health status, breeding, contraception or neutering, worming, diet, training, microchipping, pet insurance status, and indeed any problems that are arising.

Nutrition clinics

Veterinary nurses are becoming very knowledgeable about the nutritional needs of small animals from hamsters, tortoises and rabbits through to dogs. It is much more logical for them to use their time to discuss nutrition with owners than for the vet to devote precious consultation or operating time to this. Specific clinics held for several clients at a time seem to work for some practices for say overweight dogs, but in my experience, nutritional problems are usually highly individual.

If a practice is large enough to employ a VN full time as a health adviser or similar role, it becomes simpler. A nurse consulting room is designated, furnished accordingly, and the VN is allocated space on the appointment system. Referrals to this nurse come from two sources – the vets and the receptionists, and eventually from other satisfied clients. Indeed this is a logical extension of the pre-vaccination health check idea. In many practices a general health or feeding enquiry will result in a free appointment being made with this nurse. There will be practices, however, where the time of this valuable practice member will be chargeable and this is a logical progression.

A great opportunity exists for the vets in a practice to refer many cases to such a nurse after the medical consultation, either immediately or later by appointment. Examples would be the overweight dog spotted at the annual health check or with lameness problems, pets with bladder calculi or struvite problems, postoperative nutrition, diets for medical conditions, senior diets, etc. Provided he or she is properly trained and briefed, this nurse will give sound advice under much more relaxing conditions than the vet.

Once a diet regime has been implemented, this nurse can keep track of the pet's weight and condition, referring the patient back to the vet for further examinations as needed.

In smaller practices, the same ideas can easily be incorporated into the rota, and will be valuable in that common goal of practice expansion.

Dental checks

It seems to be generally held that dental tartar and periodontal disease is the great unrecognised epidemic in dogs and cats. Certainly unknown to many owners, many animals need dental attention. It seems good common sense for the vet to examine the teeth at the time of the annual health check and vaccination, but also for the practice to follow up dentistry with free dental checks. A qualified VN is eminently capable of checking the mouth for odour, plaque and tartar, and even resorption lesions and caries. Cases needing attention are referred to the vet, but the nurse is able to demonstrate teeth cleaning, give general dietary and chewing aid advice, and sell the necessary products. It would seem totally logical to emulate the dental profession and encourage twice yearly dental health checks in this way. In our experience clients wish their pets to have healthy mouths and to retain their teeth to a ripe old age, and value the advice given out at these checks. On quite a few occasions the client will mention some other problem that has been worrying them, giving the nurse the opportunity to make them an appointment with their vet.

Other possibilities

Senior health checks
As dogs and cats become older, it is quite sensible for a practice member, possibly a veterinary nurse, to check them over say, twice a year. This check might include weight, dentition, general mobility, appetite, and urine test. If any abnormalities were noted, the patient would be referred to the vet. Many owners feel comfortable with this increased frequency of health check to give them peace of mind.

Diabetic clinics
We find it useful for the owner of a diabetic dog or cat to have a daily appointment for a few days with a nurse to monitor their ability to collect and test the urine. It also is an opportunity for the nurse to train the owner in injection techniques, and for the owner to practise under supervision. The owner gains confidence much more rapidly with this sort of continuity.

Postoperative clinics
In a busy practice, nurses can be usefully employed in the release of patients after surgery or hospitalisation, re-dressings after operations, and removal of sutures. Their knowledge of dietary needs in these circumstances is also valuable.

Chapter 9
The Veterinary Surgeon
John Bower

The need to practise quality veterinary medicine and surgery is a fundamental requirement for a successful practice. Our clients entrust us with the care of their pets and assume that we are competent and up to date with modern techniques and treatments. For our part, we should ensure that we keep up with the advances in veterinary science by attendance at continuing education courses, congresses and, of course, by taking advantage of the available literature, discussions, computer programs, and videos.

The reputation of the practice will be enhanced by results, but equally by the ability or willingness of individual veterinary surgeons to discuss pets' problems with clients. By being approachable, the veterinary surgeon will ensure that the consultation is an unstressful event for clients and one that clients are happy to repeat on any occasion when they have the slightest worry about their pet. This approachable attitude is an essential requirement for practice growth and applies to the three main expansion areas, increasing the clientele, a more frequent attendance by existing clients and the expansion of services on offer.

The special situations within the practice where the veterinary surgeon can demonstrate approachability and understanding are in the consulting room, at postoperative release, on the telephone and during the euthanasia consultation.

The consulting room

The consulting room, from the practice expansion view, is the most important room in the practice. Regardless of the number of intricate surgical procedures carried out in the operating theatre, it is in the consulting room that most client–veterinarian interchanges take place. It is here that about 80% of the day's work occurs in terms of numbers of cases and it is in the consulting room that reputations are built or destroyed.

There are many rules which should be adhered to in the consulting room, and I will try to identify them.

- Consult in a clean, smart clinical coat and wear a name badge or, preferably the name and title, with the practice logo embroidered on the uniform so that the client can easily read it; for example 'Melanie Simmonds – Veterinary nurse'.
- Always remember that in the consulting room you have two patients – the pet and the owner. Each needs treating with care.

- Think of the pet as a member of the owner's family and your approach to his health and welfare will be correct.
- If the patient is already under treatment always ensure that you are familiar with the case before entering the room. This may take only a few seconds' recollection if a solo veterinary practice or a detailed perusal of the case history if a multi-man practice.
- If the case has been seen by another colleague within the practice, let the client know that you understand the case history.
- Always greet both the owner and the patient by name on entering the room, this shows the client that you 'know' them and are familiar with and concerned about the case.
- Be thorough with case history taking. I often delay the clinical examination for some minutes while I extract a full case history from the client. This may actually shorten the consultation and also serve to settle the client and pet into the consultation.
- However minor the problem, be equally thorough with your clinical examination. Apart from increasing job satisfaction, reducing the chances of misdiagnosis and justifying your consultation fee, many other unconnected problems can be noticed at this time such as dental and skin problems, cysts and tumours. It is also a useful opportunity to discuss worming and other parasite control, and may lead to future work and benefit both the patient and the practice. At no time is this more important than on the occasion of the annual health check and booster vaccinations – and it is wise to tell the clients of the benefit of the health check as well as the vaccination.
- If unsure of the diagnosis, do not be afraid to tell the client; but always indicate that you intend to identify the problem by further investigation, consultation with a colleague, or the patient's response to treatment.
- Never tell the client that they are wasting your time – even the most minor problems cause great worry to clients and in private practice if clients are prepared to pay your fee you should be prepared to alleviate their fears gently.
- Explain diagnosis, treatments, actions and prognosis. Clients like to know what is going on and increased media coverage has led to a greater awareness of surgery and medicine by the general public. In addition we should always be prepared to give an estimate for any treatment we are recommending and, if it is likely to be expensive, we should indeed offer guidelines as to probable cost even if this information is unsolicited.
- Do not hurry. On these occasions things are missed, the patient is invariably more difficult to examine if he senses that the veterinary surgeon is tense, and clients rightly feel they have not received value for money. Consultations are not necessarily shorter due to haste.
- In my opinion it is a mistake to assume the client is able to diagnose and prognose, and it is far better practice to reexamine the patient and

reassess the case after a course of treatment. The client will normally be pleased if the veterinary surgeon, at this subsequent examination, pronounces the patient healthy. As with human health, many owners prefer us to check their animals and sign them off with a clean bill of health. Provided a thorough clinical examination has been carried out, clients, in my experience, accept that a further fee is due for this consultation.

☐ With some patients, especially the elderly, periodic health checks are of benefit – to the pet, the owner and the practice.

☐ For example, assessment can be made of cardiac function, joints, dentition, anal sacs and weight. All these show continued care and interest in the patient and although not required by all clients, are welcomed by the majority of caring owners.

☐ Try to find time to discuss the clients' other interests in life – family, local football, obedience training, etc. – if needed note these briefly on the client's records. We often find ourselves these days as substitutes for the family doctor in terms of discussing problems and providing contact.

Postoperative release

The postoperative release consultation is a rather special one and should be treated as such. All of the foregoing applies and it is a valuable occasion on which to demonstrate both skill and a caring attitude. However minor the procedure, the client will almost certainly have been worried all day. If time allows, the veterinary surgeon should grasp the opportunity to discuss first hand what has been done and the likely outcome – this emphasises that the patient is an individual and not just a number. Postoperative care should be outlined and in addition a printed instruction sheet is useful to remind the client of your verbal instructions.

On the telephone

It is, of course, essential to have an efficient but polite, perceptive, knowledgeable and helpful filter system around the veterinary surgeon to prevent unnecessary involvement in telephone conversations with clients. The employment of veterinary nurses has in recent years meant that many queries can be dealt with competently without the involvement of the veterinarian, but where the receptionist or nurse feels that the client should speak to a veterinary surgeon, or the client insists, then it is sound business sense to do so. If you are too busy to speak to the client, they may well call someone who is not.

The telephone conversation must be productive and of use to the client. This is not the time to be harassed, angry, or short of time at the start of the conversation. Imagine yourself in the reverse role with, say, the doctor, or a hotelier. Consumers like using people with whom they can communicate. Many telephone conversations can end up with advice to present the patient at the surgery. The consultation so generated ensures that the pet receives the best possible treatment while the client feels that he or she has been looked after. The resultant consultation fee is expected and accepted and the client invariably leaves the surgery satisfied – a feeling that they communicate to their friends and acquaintances.

However, dissatisfaction at the outcome of this telephone call will not result in a consultation but an even more talkative client whose comments will adversely affect the practice.

Laboratory tests

An area where the telephone is perhaps underused is that of the laboratory test result. Increasingly, laboratory and other aids to diagnosis are being used and the corresponding fees charged. The client should be informed as soon as the test result is known. It is all too easy to make a note on the patient records for your own use and then to charge the client who feels the fee is unjustified as they are not aware of the benefit of the test. Very few clients object to paying for such an aid to diagnosis provided they are told of its use and significance in the case. Communicating the result to the client shows you are following the case closely. Remember that a result showing all is normal will alleviate unwarranted fears. This again is an opportunity to demonstrate to the client that their case is under constant review.

The euthanasia consultation

One of the most important occasions on which a veterinary surgeon can demonstrate understanding is when called upon to euthanase a much loved family pet. At no other time are the qualities of caring and understanding more required. Owners at this time are highly emotional and extremely sensitive to the attitude of the veterinary surgeon (and nurse) in attendance. Euthanasia carried out with appropriate consideration for the pet and owner will win many new clients by word of mouth recommendation for the practice – whereas the converse also applies. It is the one occasion on which I feel the wishes of the owner should be paramount – they should be allowed to decide whether the pet is euthanased in his own surroundings at home, or in the surgery and also whether they wish to be present or not. The veterinary surgeon should fit in with their wishes.

Guidelines for euthanasia

I recommend the following guidelines for euthanasia in the home.

❏ Always ensure that the owner is convinced that the euthanasia is necessary.

❐ Handle the pet with gentleness and understanding. Remember that he is in most cases regarded as one of the owner's family.

❐ Encourage the owner to be present.

❐ Explain the procedure.

❐ Explain exactly what will (and may) happen.

❐ The procedure must be smooth for the pet and the owner, whatever the sacrifice in terms of time.

❐ Remember to get the consent form signed.

❐ The pet will often be on a sofa, bed, or floor, and the vet should perform the euthanasia in this position if possible.

❐ The owner or nurse should hold the pet and raise the vein.

❐ Ensure the pet lies in the sleeping position afterwards when the dose takes effect.

❐ Do expect, and indeed encourage, tears at this moment. Grieving is normal.

❐ Sympathise: say what a peaceful end when the time had come.

❐ Warn of the possibility of nervous signs.

❐ Accept any offer of a cup of tea – or suggest it – and talk!

❐ Caringly discuss the disposal of the body and outline the alternatives.

❐ If asked to leave the body behind, enquire if you can carry it anywhere for the owner.

❐ If requested to take the body away, it may be better to suggest that the owner leaves the room while the body is placed in the plastic bag. No owner wants to be present to see that, and it may be more acceptable to wrap the body in a blanket.

❐ Carry the body in your arms caringly and place it carefully and gently in the car. Be aware that the grieving owner will often be watching from the front window to see how you handle their deceased pet at this stage.

❐ Having placed the body in the car, return to the house under the pretext of washing your hands to have a final reassuring chat with the owner.

The same general principles also apply in the surgery but extra consideration must be given to the owner when the euthanasia is completed. Try to have a member of staff available to give support to the distressed owner; a cup of tea may not go unappreciated. Where possible have a separate exit from the surgery so that grief-stricken owners do not have to walk out past waiting clients.

Payment for euthanasia is always a delicate subject. Some clients prefer to pay at the time so that they do not receive reminders of the pet through the post later, while others are so shaken that they need to leave the premises as quickly as possible.

An added note of caution here: nothing upsets a client more than a booster reminder card sent for a deceased pet so if your computer records system does not automatically delete reminders for deceased patients, ensure your staff routinely remove reminder cards from the file when pets are euthanased.

If the pet and/or client is well known to your practice, a sympathetic note of condolence from you a few days later will be well received.

If euthanasia is handled properly your next task may well be to vaccinate a new puppy or kitten.

Chapter 10
Staff Motivation
John Bower

Motivate your staff and your practice will become happier and more successful. Motivate means to 'supply a motive', i.e., a positive act on the part of the employer to give the members of staff a reason to want the practice to be successful – to feel part of the team; to feel it is 'our' not 'your' practice.

We are all consumers – our clients no more or less than ourselves. Whether we like it or not we are a professional equivalent of, say, a restaurant. There is surely no real difference between the reasons why clients come to a particular practice and why we like to eat in a particular restaurant – for the welcome, the pleasant willing service and the product. It is quite noticeable that successful restaurants, i.e., the busy ones, depend on the people 'fronting' them and serving the customers. The same guidelines apply to creating and maintaining a successful veterinary practice; no matter how good you are, your staff are equally important.

Staff motivation starts with selecting the staff – employing the right type of person for the position within the practice. This is never more necessary than with the position of receptionist which is arguably the most important post within the practice. The receptionist may have no other function or may also be a nurse or may indeed be one of several who are expected to answer the telephone or doorbell. Receptionists must be people who like people – if they like animals as well that is a bonus. They must also be sympathetic and caring to enable them to deal with people with problems. Most people who consult us have a problem and this may come over as anger or impatience. The receptionist must recognise this and react accordingly.

For the practice to grow, the client must telephone the practice or come into it first and then if they like what they see, they must be convinced to use the practice again, and again. But if they are put off on that initial telephone contact, they will not come in any more than one would with difficult receptionists in other businesses.

The same attitudes must apply to all other members of the practice who come into contact with the clients. So how do you ensure that staff become possessive about and intimately involved in the practice?

First, of course, everyone in the practice should be convinced that the practice produces good quality veterinary medicine and surgery, and does so in a caring fashion. They have to see fair play. It is quite reasonable to charge the correct fee for routine work and it is quite reasonable to reduce this fee for children's pets, cases that are going on longer than perhaps anticipated or for pets owned by senior citizens. It is unreasonable to charge anyone for treatment of small wild creatures brought in for help during normal working hours.

The caring attitude must extend to a willingness to provide the obligatory 24 hour service to urgent cases, whatever the time of day or night. Conversely, staff should be respected and backed up when they are being unfairly criticised.

Having obtained the respect of the staff for work and service, it is necessary to make them feel important within the practice structure. This could include identifying them within the practice – smart uniforms with name badges for veterinary nurses, perhaps different uniforms (outfits chosen by them) for receptionists, again with name badges, and encouragement for the veterinary surgeons to wear clean presentable clinical coats or jackets when consulting, by either providing these garments or at least laundering them on the practice.

Status and individuality are also given to the practice personnel by listing their names, position and qualifications on a separate notice board in the reception area or waiting room. Smart, glass framed display boards with interchangeable lettering are available from office equipment suppliers and stationers.

Pay is, of course, important, but not necessarily always the most important aspect. It is very necessary to pay a fair wage but oddly enough if all of the other 'motivators' are attended to, the actual pay becomes less important. That is, it becomes less important to pay the highest wage possible.

Recognition of tasks well done or of the ability of a certain member of staff is all important. Ensure you compliment someone who has done a good job whether it be a surgical procedure, a particularly clean and tidy consulting room or a clean ward. Staff achievements should not be taken for granted. If a member of staff has had a particularly good year for one reason or another, why not a cash bonus, for instance?

Promotion

The concept of promotion or advancement within the practice should be carefully thought out, both in terms of pay and responsibility. This will apply both to the nursing staff who may progress from student veterinary nurse to head nurse, and to professional staff from assistant veterinary surgeon, through senior assistant or salaried partner to full partner. The increased responsibility that attaches to this promotion is a great motivator. Employed staff like responsibility so delegation is a motivator and also takes the pressure off you. Thus you motivate the head nurse who motivates student nurses, etc. Let the staff, for instance, work out their own on and off duty rota with a proviso that there must always be somebody on duty and available. This applies mainly to nurses but could also apply to assistants. The facility for staff to participate in and make decisions on their own rota will also lead to a greater feeling of being part of a team.

It is this concept of teamwork that is the single most important factor within a successful practice. The atmosphere within that practice must be one of happy teamwork. This rapidly transmits to attending clients who also therefore feel happy. Any disgruntlements or frictions within the practice should be discussed at an early stage before they have a chance to grow out of proportion. I regret to say that if there is an obvious odd man out within the practice, steps must be taken to sort out the problem or dismiss that person for the good of everyone concerned.

An essential part of feeling one of the team is participation in running the practice. Staff involvement in decisions and the running of systems within the practice could be implemented. I thoroughly recommend staff meetings. These can be held out of normal hours, possibly within the practice premises and involving only members of staff. Such meetings are of course, a genuine practice expense so why not have a little wine and encourage everyone to have their say. These meetings are invaluable but should not be held too frequently or they become grumbling sessions. Perhaps two or three times a year is ideal.

Another team building exercise is to have practice socials from time to time. The Christmas dinner, held one evening a week or so before Christmas, is an eagerly anticipated social event – by both employees and employers alike. It is held in a local bistro which provides a private room and proves a great leveller. Only current practice members are invited and the food, wine, conversation and camaraderie flows. In recent years, we have hired a DJ and invited spouses to join in after the meal.

Throughout the year skittle evenings, cinema trips, summer barbecues, etc., are all enthusiastically attended, and organised by the support staff and practice manager. We regard these functions as essential team builders and they certainly aid cohesion within the practice.

A recent idea which seems to work in the USA, is the so-called 'retreat' where practice members are treated to a short weekend away at a hotel cum leisure centre. This is a structured weekend with talks on most of the topics covered in this section of the book, sometimes with guest speakers, and an evening social and dinner. I am certain the idea has merit.

This then is the answer – communication. And it must be a two way thing. Staff must know for instance the pathways for complaints or grievances, that is which partner deals with their problems. If so requested, that partner must set time aside to talk. All practices should have a room available for private discussion or interviews. Pent-up working frustration leads to apathy, resistance to change, aggression or regression, all destructive and infectious tendencies within a practice.

It is essential, of course, to give the staff the right instructions, advice and training and then to have a facility for ensuring that they understand and communicate, for instance, practice policies. It must be explained to

raw young student nurses or indeed veterinary assistants why it is necessary to smile and be pleasant.

Continuing professional development (CPD) within the practice should
be taken seriously. Fees spent on sending an assistant to a BSAVA/C-Vet
clinical weekend, national congress or local meeting will be well rewarded
by the information and enthusiasm brought back to the practice.

Comprehensive notes should be requested so the whole practice benefits. Why not also hang the framed certificate of attendance in your
waiting room alongside degree certificates or further qualifications? The
nursing staff should be treated equally.

These attendances at continuing education courses can and should be
mentioned to clients. Indeed any opportunity to inform clients of the
capabilities of staff should be grasped, as it reinforces the feeling of
importance in the practice of those concerned and it shows the client that
you are a progressive practice.

Bonus schemes are applicable in staff motivation, as already discussed;
but provided all other working conditions are good, a fair salary which is
a reflection of the value of the individual within the practice is usually
appreciated. However, an 'out of hours' bonus scheme is recommended so
that work during antisocial hours is rewarded.

In general, the successful practice will have a family atmosphere
(whether the staff number three or forty), and will be a welcoming place
for clients and their pets. It will be thought of as important in the local
community and held in high regard, will be seen as socially responsible in
its approach to treatment of wildlife, children's and pensioners' pets and
those of the financially handicapped – and everyone in the practice should
be made to feel that they are an important part of this valuable service to
the community.

Chapter 11
Staff Training

John Bower

Training, both initial and ongoing, is as important to the team development as obtaining the right staff to start with using in-depth and consistent interviewing. It is a great mistake, and one I am sure we have all made, to employ the right person, explain a little about the task, then leave them to it, and grumble or dismiss them when they don't come up to expectation.

Training will consist of a combination of:

❐ instruction in specific, technical matters
❐ guidance in non-technical people skills which build the employee's ability to work with other members of the team, and also to communicate and cope with the general public
❐ specific training in practice protocols, the vision and aims of the practice – in other words the ethos of the practice, which may be well understood and entrenched in the long term staff but baffling or even quite foreign to a new member who has worked in a very different sort of practice, another profession, or who may have never been in paid employment before.

It is important that new members of staff learn the practices and procedures as quickly as possible, so that they become part of the team in the shortest possible time. A structured induction programme achieves this and also reduces the level of anxiety naturally felt by anyone joining a new employer. A reasonable induction period may last approximately six weeks. During that time the new employee should initially 'shadow' someone carrying out the tasks for which they will be expected to be responsible. The person they shadow may vary from day to day or week to week but should always be the best and most appropriate person for that phase of the new employee's in-house training. Ideally, for example, a new student veterinary nurse (SVN) may start working in the ward alongside a qualified veterinary nurse (VN) who is not only competent at her job but is able to convey enthusiasm and communicate effectively with the new employee. He or she may spend five half days in the ward area of the hospital learning about in-patient care as we want it to be, but also learns record keeping, use of ward sheets, use of the computer for clinical records, instructions and pricing, and communication with other key members of staff such as vets in charge of ward cases.

The 'trainer' should impress on the new employee the essential nature of good, regular communication with owners of hospitalised patients, the visiting policy, and what to do when owners ask questions which the SVN is not qualified to answer. The new SVN may spend the other five half days in the reception area learning what it is like at the sharp end of the client–practice interface, how a good receptionist answers the phone, deals with queries, makes appointments, handles the fee aspect with clients, communicates with other practice members, greets and empathises with clients, and is generally essential to the business and smooth running of the practice.

Other areas new staff should be familiar with are the laboratory, prep. room, dispensary, office, and consulting rooms. Being present and helping in some consulting sessions with one of the vets gives more insight as to how the practice works and the relationship between the practice and its clients. In each area the new person should be encouraged to ask questions, be shown exactly how things are done, not be made to feel stupid if they ask for their trainer to repeat something, and their confidence should be slowly built in order for them to start functioning as rapidly as possible as a useful team member. In our experience it is far more fruitful to make haste slowly, and to ensure simple tasks are completed thoroughly and well before moving on to more complex tasks and overfacing the individual so that they become anxious or begin making mistakes.

By the end of the six week induction period the new member should have a thorough understanding of how all parts of the practice fit together and how they as a 'cog' in that mechanism are essential to its smooth functioning. The new employee should be reasonably competent at carrying out essential tasks, and have shown the ability and enthusiasm for learning much more. Helping the person to become effective, developing a strong interest in doing their job well, having role models to teach good practice and learning that good work is appreciated and recognised will all help. It is also important during this induction phase that the new member is recognised as an individual, that every one else talks to them about common interests e.g. hobbies and makes them feel welcome not *just* as another student.

After six weeks carry out a short induction appraisal (see Chapter 12). In a small minority of cases it may become apparent after the induction period that this job is not going to be suitable for them or that they are not best fitted to the tasks. If that is the case it may be better to cut your losses, admit you have both made a mistake at interview and part before any more time or effort is wasted for both parties.

A comprehensive practice manual (see Chapter 17) is an excellent way of communicating the basics, and eliminates the need for these procedures to be outlined laboriously whenever a new member joins. It is obvious, however, that the induction programme for new staff will vary – for a secretary, the programme will be different from that for a veterinarian, or a new receptionist or student nurse.

Ongoing training then needs to be monitored by the senior vet, practice manager, or head of that department, depending on the size and shape of your practice. Clinical training and development should never be static as this leads to stagnation and boredom. Student nurse training is well structured under the NVQ umbrella, but vets and qualified nurses can work towards certificates, diplomas or health counselling qualification and must be encouraged to remain up to date on all aspects of their work. Forward thinking practices will budget a CPD allowance for their staff. In addition receptionists and office personnel should be encouraged to attend training courses which improve their skills, provided they are matched to the practice's needs. For example improved computer or accounting skills may be required in the office, or a receptionist may feel she needs help with her management of difficult clients or stress or both.

We have found it useful to run regular in-house training sessions for the whole practice team to discuss non-clinical topics such as pet health insurance, marketing practice services and customer care. These may take the form of a one hour session led by an appropriate member of the team or a whole day session led by a trainer from outside the practice. Although the training can consist of presentations and talks, role playing is a great help in illustrating vividly the difference between a good and bad approach to the client, and in working relationships with other team members.

Chapter 12
Staff Appraisals

John Bower

Staff appraisals should not be linked to, or combined with salary reviews – these should be separate items. The most successful appraisal includes an element of self assessment in advance of the meeting, and then a comparison of the employee's and employers' comments and opinions. This leads naturally into a discussion as to how things can be improved, and indeed rarely do the opinions differ. The assessment should have no vindictive aim at all, but rather work on the concept of emphasising the good points and identifying a few areas where more work or effort is needed. Clarify at the outset what the appraisal is all about, work hard at avoiding the staff getting the wrong impression and take care to present the process as a means of:

- ❐ learning from the past to aid the future
- ❐ recognising abilities and potential
- ❐ developing knowledge, skills and attitudes
- ❐ building on successes and overcoming difficulties
- ❐ increasing motivation and job satisfaction
- ❐ enhancing relationships and furthering team work.

Plan the appraisal thoroughly and address the basic questions of *why*, *who*, *where*, *when*, *what*, and *how* in readiness for a 'meeting of minds'. In fact everyone involved should give it advance thought. It should be a collaborative venture between management and staff as one-sided planning tends to give a one-sided discussion and one-sided outcome.

Appraisals should never be treated as an interview but as a discussion, and above all they must be positive. An appointment time is set by the appraiser, giving the appraisee about two weeks notice. Set this time so that cancellation is avoided, barring dire emergencies. It can take place during the working day in a quiet room in the practice, or even away from it if necessary. Put a sign on the door to ensure you are not interrupted and stress that neither of you should be called to answer the phone. It is essential that the process is seen as important, personal and confidential. Any personal and private facts revealed within the appraisal should stay private, but may be noted on that person's personal record if appropriate and if agreed. It is essential that trust is established and maintained throughout this process.

Actions agreed upon as a result of the appraisal will become more public, depending on their nature.

Who appraises whom?

In a small practice, the principal will probably carry out all the appraisals, and if he or she is brave enough, ask another senior practice member to appraise him. In a larger practice, appraisals can be delegated. For example the head nurse could appraise the nursing staff, and could in turn be appraised by, say, the practice manager or partners. The practice manager will probably be appraised by a partner. What about the partners? Appraisal should not stop here – each partner should be appraised by another partner or another senior member of staff. This I feel is a valuable move in the practice. A note of caution – training in conducting appraisals is available and highly recommended before embarking on this very important role.

Types of appraisal

In our practice we have three main types of appraisal:

❐   induction appraisals
❐   mini appraisals
❐   full appraisals.

The induction appraisal
This is conducted at the end of the six week induction period for a new member of staff.

It is an informal chat taking about 30 minutes and is to find out how the new member of the practice feels they are doing, identify any problem areas, and help to guide them towards becoming a full member of the practice team. It is an opportunity for the appraiser to assess whether the appraisee has understood the ethos of the practice, their role and to ensure they are still fully committed to staying and progressing. Brief notes may be kept, signed and filed in the employee's personal folder.

The mini appraisal
The mini appraisal can look at:

❐   how the job is going
❐   how the staff member is doing or if there are problems
❐   how can they develop
❐   what can be done to make it happen.

The purpose of a mini appraisal is to allow open but confidential communication, and prevent any problems that may arise from escalating for the sake of 'a good chat' or clearing of the air. Their regularity will vary – some team members seem to need or want frequent mini appraisals, whilst others hardly ever do.

The full appraisal

This may take 1–2 hours and again it is essential that adequate warning is given, forms filled in by both parties, and time set aside and kept to for this process. We conduct full appraisals on an annual basis, using a team of senior staff members who have received training in conducting appraisals. This means that each of us is allocated a small number of appraisees each and we work gradually through their appraisals at times which are mutually convenient.

Each appraisal should be conducted with both parties having knowledge and preferably a copy of the practice business objectives. The reason for this is that the appraisee's objectives can be matched as closely as possible to those of the practice, with convergence of effort and aims. For example one practice objective may be to target the exotics market more effectively, and during an appraisal an individual may express a great interest in this area. Conversely, someone may wish to go on an IT course which they would find most interesting but would have less relevance to the needs of the practice in their position.

Examples of some of the questions asked on the appraisal form are shown in Fig. 12.1. There should be no big surprises if team members know each other and work together, and generally we find that there is broad agreement in answers to all questions on the appraisal form. It is important to allow time for discussion where necessary without labouring points, and for the appraiser to let the appraisee do most of the talking. It is a very positive experience to have a senior member of staff giving you their undivided attention in this way, but it must never be allowed to turn into a moaning session. Appraisees should be encouraged to suggest their own solutions for any problems identified, rather than laying them at your

---

Preparation for appraisal (employee self-assessment)

(A)   The job

(1)   What are the main tasks or responsibilities in your job?

(2)   Which areas of your work do you think have gone particularly well in the last six months or so? Also why did those go particularly well?

(3)   Which areas of your work have proved particularly difficult? Again why do you think this is?

(4)   How would you anticipate your job could develop or otherwise change over the next year? Prioritise if necessary.

Continued on facing page

Continued from previous page

(B) Work partnerships

(1) At work, which member(s) of the team most directly affects the way you perform your job?

(2) Which people at work are most directly affected by the way you perform your job?

(3) At work, what support and assistance do you receive from others?

(4) At work, what support and assistance do you give others?

(5) How would you like to see your working relationships change or develop over the next year?

(C) This veterinary practice and you

(1) How do you feel in general terms about working with this veterinary practice? Please detail things about this practice and its work about which you feel particularly happy or unhappy.

(2) How do you see your future with this practice? Please detail any particular aspirations and ambitions you have.

(D) Other aspects

(1) Are there any other points you would like to raise that haven't been covered so far?

(E) Ideas for action

(1) What would you like to see done to help with the items indicated in Sections (A), (B), (C) and (D)?

(2) What could you do to help things along?

Figure 12.1 Example of an assessment form.

feet and expecting you to go away and sort their difficulties out for them. A well structured appraisal form encourages this approach. Often very useful initiatives arise from lateral discussions during appraisals, and junior members of the team are able to make equally positive contributions towards ideas for the smooth running of the practice as older or more long term staff. In fact new staff may see things in new and original ways.

The main points discussed in the appraisal and any actions agreed to be taken forward to the practice manager or partners are written up, signed and dated by both parties.

Regular appraisals help the practice team enormously. They help in the development of staff skills and roles, they prevent the continuance of bad habits, and can sort out differences in aims and objectives. In the absence of regular appraisals, an invitation to 'see the boss' invariably means a confrontation, a difficult interview. If an appraisal is imminent, then the same needed interview becomes a discussion with a different, positive attitude, and the whole practice benefits.

Chapter 13
Interview Techniques
John Bower

As a successful practice expands, more staff will be needed to carry out the increased work load. Practice attitudes, policies and services should not change for the worse with the introduction and training of new members of the practice. Teamwork is central to the success of a progressive practice so the correct selection of veterinary surgeons, receptionists and nurses is essential.

Thus the interview, all important to the applicant, should be taken equally seriously by the employer and planned well ahead. This is by no means commonplace, and many of us are guilty of giving an interview no forethought whatsoever, asking whatever questions come into our minds in a totally unplanned fashion, and making our minds up within two to five minutes of the start of the interview. True, this 'snap' judgement may give an indication of whether the applicant is a person that we can 'get on with' but whether or not they are suitable for the task in hand is a matter of luck.

An essential ingredient of planning ahead is to request from each applicant a curriculum vitae (CV) which should cover personal details, education, history, seeing practice experience, management experience (did new graduates attend the SPVS/BVA first postgraduate job management symposium?), interests and special skills and, importantly, references. These references would not normally be taken up at this stage but become much more relevant if consideration is being given to employing the applicant after a formal interview.

Much can be gained from a structured interview and there is a lot to be said for asking the same questions of each applicant so a direct comparison can be drawn. It is the interviewer's role to make the applicant feel at ease as this will ensure a more fruitful interview. A relaxed, friendly approach, informal seating positions in an office, over a cup of coffee perhaps, is preferable to the intimidating situation of the classic interview where the applicant is a lonely figure on a chair on one side of the desk with the interviewer(s) lined up on the other side. A two to three minute settling-in period over general conversation while the interviewer assesses the attitude and dress of the applicant (and vice versa) is a useful start. To an applicant this attention to dress may seem irrelevant but to a veterinary surgeon, about to integrate new personnel in to the team, it may well be all important.

Preliminary questions

It is sensible to ask a few direct questions first with yes, no answers. Such questions could include 'Have you a driving licence, a criminal record, or any disability which prevents you from carrying out work which may involve anaesthesia, X-rays, lifting heavy dogs, or handling farm animals?' If you have a small staff room and smoking is a problem, it is sensible to ask if the applicant is a non-smoker. Anyone looking for an excuse to employ non-smokers should look to a recent survey in the USA which demonstrated that smokers are 20% more expensive to employ due to illness, accidents involving fire, and smoking breaks (D. McCurnin, personal communication). At this stage it would be worth asking if there are any complications with the applicant's life style that would make it difficult to fulfil 24-hour on call obligations or working overtime if necessary.

Having disposed of these few yes, no answers, the rest of the interview should consist of open ended questions so that the applicant is made to sell him/herself. Far too many interviews consist of the interviewers interviewing themselves, answering questions put by a fellow partner, or talking of practice policies and justifying them at an inappropriate stage of the interview.

Many potential questions concerning education, job experience, interests and hobbies will have been covered by the CV but some may be worth expanding. Certainly work habits, likes and dislikes, and hard held principles can be legitimately extracted. An interesting and often fruitful line is to ask what motivates the applicant and conversely which parts of the job, if any, are less tolerable. An interesting insight can develop. It may be useful to know the short term and long term personal goals of the applicant especially as they relate to the position being offered. In addition, it is very important to know why the applicant is attracted to the post on offer and, indeed, what skills or benefits they will bring with them to the practice. A poser which sometimes produces surprising answers is to ask what is the applicant's greatest achievement so far in their life?

There is never a better time to set down ground rules than at an interview. Now is the time to state whether the post offered is for a trial period or permanent and to ask how the applicant feels about constructive criticism or a formal evaluation of his or her work after a set period.

It is of great importance to ascertain if the interviewee will fit in with the practice team whether as a veterinary surgeon, nurse or receptionist. Thus a useful question to ask would be 'How were you treated at your previous employment? Were you happy that you received the encouragement or recognition that you deserved?' It may be then easier to assess whether that person would integrate or would have the same grievances within one's own practice.

Proof of literacy and mathematical ability may be required, although, for a veterinary surgeon, gaining the degree should provide proof of both. However, a short (100 word) statement, handwritten, on some aspect of veterinary work, views on 24-hour call or a statement on some aspect of animal welfare may provide this proof along with a useful insight into personal views. A simple calculation on dosages of medicines for animals of certain weights using certain concentrations (a frequent problem in practice) will show a basic grasp of maths for a potential nurse or receptionist.

Interaction

We like to prolong any interview to give the applicant time to wander around the practice at will, after introductions, and talk to any member of staff. Apart from genuinely giving the applicant a chance to probe potential team mates about what we are really like, a consensus of opinion about the applicant develops which is most useful in the final selection. In addition, we will often encourage a fellow staff member to take the applicant out to lunch if we wish to obtain an extra viewpoint. Our interviews tend to vary in length from all day or even longer if possible for veterinary surgeons, to several hours or a day for receptionists and nurses coupled with a day actively involved, if on the short list. All this is aimed at reducing the chances of employing personnel who just do not fit in to the practice team for one reason or another.

References, usually listed on the CV, are all important and in my opinion should always be taken up for applicants who are about to be offered the job. It is worth probing below the surface of the bland pleasant reference with searching questions that reveal whether your perceptions of the applicant are correct, what are their work habits, what motivates them and how was their standing in the practice. Question the reason given for leaving and always ask the definitive question 'Would you employ them again if they were available?'

Exit interview

Conversely, when an employee leaves your practice voluntarily, always take time to carry out an exit interview on the very last day of employment to find out the genuine reason they are leaving and what problems they see in the practice. Valuable information can be gained at this time only and if this information is used, it can be of great benefit to the practice.

Chapter 14
Partners' Responsibilities

Dixon Gunn

The smallest possible veterinary practice contains one veterinary surgeon and an electronic method of transferring calls; the largest practice might involve over one hundred people, as veterinary surgeons, nurses, secretaries and a host of part-time telephonists. The principles of management are the same for either extreme.

Veterinary practices may now be owned by anyone, including limited companies. This new arrangement does not vary the responsibilities of those in charge to set up a correct management structure for the benefit of both clients and staff. Therefore perhaps the title of this chapter may appear out of date but as the number of practices which have converted to corporate status, either by individual choice or by being bought, is still relatively small, it is correct to discuss 'partners' responsibilities'. This title can be extended to include directors and managers in the new framework. The actual running of the corporate practice will be delegated to senior veterinarians and senior managers. These are collectively included in the term 'partners' in this chapter.

It is useful to consider a practice as made up of several departments, not all of which may have identical aims. An explanatory example of this might be the question of the purchase of an expensive piece of equipment, e.g. an endoscope, not as a replacement but as a new venture.

The partner in charge of practice promotion is all for it, the partner in charge of finance is not, or not at this time. Putting their case to other partners helps clarify the situation and with luck an amicable agreement is reached. A principal has the same problems to face, but he has only himself to argue with. Whether this improves the quality of debate is doubtful.

The names given to the departments can be rather grand, such as 'Treasury' or 'Personnel management', but for most practices the following titles will cover the various responsibilities: personnel, finance, stock control, motor vehicles, working arrangements, fabric maintenance and promotion.

Personnel

The partner with responsibilities for personnel has an increasing remit due to the continual development of the employer–employee relationship. All employers must carry employees' liability insurance and display the appropriate certificate at each of the businesses where persons covered by the policy are employed: that is at each branch as well as at the main surgery premises.

Protection of employees and of visiting clients must be given due priority within a practice. The Health and Safety at Work Act 1974 is designed to do just what the title implies, protect the health and safety of persons in the work place, and it has wide ramifications.

The correct disposal of noxious materials, whether it be pharmaceutical waste, clinical waste or innocent household waste, must be dealt with accordingly.

RIDDOR – Reporting of Injuries, Diseases and Dangerous Occurrences Regulations 1995 is designed to take care of the correct reporting of accidents in the work place.

COSHH (Control of Substances Hazardous to Health) Regulations 1999 are of particular importance in veterinary practice with potent medicines, inflammable and caustic materials.

Members of staff under the age of 18 must not be involved in the taking of X-rays. Women of child-bearing age must be made aware of the risks of radiation, of contact with certain gaseous anaesthetics and some veterinary medicines, as well as disease risks.

One way of addressing these potential problems is to have a Standard Operating Procedure (SOP) written out for each circumstance. SOPs should be short, written in simple language and address the following points.

❐ Who may carry out the procedure?
❐ How it is to be done?
❐ Where and when it may be undertaken?

A good start is to have the first draft written by the person who is currently undertaking the procedure.

Hopefully all these precautions remain as warnings. The more important day to day responsibility of the partner in charge of personnel is overseeing the working arrangements of staff and being identified as the partner to whom queries are taken, possibly through a chain of command, from trainee nurse to head nurse to partner. He or she should also prepare for and be present at interviews of prospective employees. Staff appraisals, if undertaken by the practice, also fall within this busy remit.

Job satisfaction is often linked to continued training and, as and when appropriate, the partner responsible should be involved in overseeing the training of junior members of staff and in promoting opportunities for more senior members to continue their professional development. A practice training schedule with a budget attached is the modern approach.

Staff comfort covers numerous items such as appropriate uniforms, facilities for coffee and lunch breaks and, of high significance, payment of wages on time.

At the end of this first section there are two points to make which cover all partnership responsibilities. First, despite the long list of jobs within the department, the partner in charge does not have to carry out each one himself. The bigger the practice, the greater degree of delegation that can and should be used. Second, in the ideal situation there should be at least one other person who understands and can take over any given job in the practice. The back-up does not have to be a partner or even a veterinary surgeon, but it has to be wrong if, because one person is sick, the computer remains silent.

Finance

Cash flow
It is essential to know the financial situation at any given time. The subject of cash flow dealt with in Chapter 26 covers the method of keeping a regular supply of finance to meet the practice requirements.

Cash flow only tells part of the story. Management accounts should be produced on a monthly basis providing the owners with significant parameters at a glance.

For example, what proportion of turnover is swallowed up as expenses? Work this out on an annual basis using the equation:

$$\frac{\text{Total expenses} \times 365}{\text{Turnover}}$$

The answer in days is comparable year on year. Alternatively total expenses can be presented as a percentage of turnover giving a figure for comparison irrespective of the time span. (See Chapter 27 Management Accounts.)

Book debt
How much is owed to the practice and how many days work does this represent? (See Chapters 23 and 29.)

Cash at bank and in hand
Partners do not have salaries, even if the practice says that they do. The 'salary' they draw is not taxed at source and is simply a drawing against expected profits. These profits have to cover the income tax payable on the year's profits, National Insurance contributions and the capital expenditure of the practice. Taking these three items into account it is as well to contemplate drawings during the year which do not exceed 50% of the final net profit figures.

The control of drawings is of paramount importance if practices are not to run into unnecessary debt with consequent expensive repayments. Monthly drawings must be agreed in advance and no more taken without the specific agreement of the partners after discussion with the partner in charge of finance. A desire to place more in a pension fund must be balanced by taking less for oneself if it is not to upset the capital structure of the practice.

Capital investment happens every year, whether as a large sum in property or a small sum in equipment. The method of funding the purchase has to be considered carefully along with the method and time of repayment, leasing versus overdraft versus available capital. One person in a practice must look at the possibilities and report to the rest.

As a very basic rule, planning to leave 10% of net profits in the practice each year will go some way towards meeting the requirement of purchasing new equipment and making necessary improvements.

Stock control

The more large animal work involved, the larger is this department in the practice. Drug purchase in mixed practice is the biggest single item of expenditure, accounting for some 30% of turnover. Careful control can improve cash flow and profits dramatically.

The level of stock on the shelves, the frequency of turnover and the ability to adjust in the face of an outbreak of a specific disease are all critical. Even more important is routine checking of invoices which should ideally arrive already priced at the same time as the delivery. Every time a consignment arrives a check should be undertaken to ensure that:

❐ the product is there in its correct amount
❐ the purchase price has not altered since the last purchase
❐ the invoice itself is correctly totalled
❐ any 'to follows' are noted.

A system of checking must be set up and understood by all personnel involved in unpacking drug supplies. This is a perfect example of the delegation required by the partner in charge of stock control. He or she is responsible while a member of support staff carries out the duty.

A missed alteration in purchase price results in a lower or negative margin on the resale of that item. It is not uncommon in farm practice to have a large order delivered for one farm, passed on and booked out on the same day (which happens to be the last day of the month) and before an increase in cost price is recognised, the account has been rendered.

Some drugs must be kept under lock and key and a record of their use made on every occasion this occurs. The key should only be available to nominated persons within the practice, but all members of staff should be aware of the legal requirements of the practice (see Chapter 20 Stock Control).

Motor vehicles

Motor vehicles may not seem to justify a department of their own but, except in purely small animal practice, they do form an important section.

Reliability of travel in adverse conditions is essential. Will the practice use diesel or lead free petrol, two or four wheel drive, buy new or second hand cars? A partner should be made responsible for monitoring the vehicles and determining when to change a car. Lease hire, hire purchase, contract leasing and straight purchase are all in the melting pot when considering how to acquire the next vehicle. It should be remembered that every method other than a straight purchase involves a third party in the transaction and that third party is there because he is being paid to be there.

Working arrangements

Rotas for support staff and professional staff and the forward booking of routine work such as meat inspection, kennel inspections, routine fertility visits, puppy clinics and weight watcher clinics fall under the 'working arrangements' title. Every practice has some of this type of commitment and planning ahead prevents the catastrophe of one veterinary surgeon being expected to be in two places at once.

The requirement to provide a 24 hour service means a rota of 'duty vets'. This overlaps with the personnel department in that there are two requirements: (1) to be fair to all in terms of their contract of employment and (2) to build in a flexibility to allow changes; missing your sister's wedding because you are on call can be a serious family black mark.

As practice becomes more specialised, the mixed practice can face difficulty in arranging out of hours cover for all the species catered for. Some veterinary surgeons are unwilling to attend emergency farm work or equine work simply because of lack of experience and an understandable fear of letting the animal, the client and the practice down. Sharing rotas with a neighbour or using the services of an emergency clinic are possible solutions to this difficult problem of providing adequate out of hours cover without upsetting the veterinary staff of the practice.

Promotion

Promotion is now a major interest of the progressive practice. The partner responsible has to be guided by his own instincts and the comments of his colleagues. Newsletters, practice brochures, information to clients by way of handouts, invitation to promotional meetings, advertising, development of PML sales in large animal work and front counter sales in small animal practice all form part of the image of the practice. The partners must decide in advance what they want their image to be.

Property maintenance should be included in this final section. It is an important item, and it has a great deal to do with practice promotion.

Every change in the face of the property is interesting to the clients. Interest by the clients is beneficial to the practice. Continual updating is essential.

Few practices have six partners to take one section each as detailed above. Irrespective of the number of people available it will be beneficial to the principal or the partners to consider each section in turn, thinking of the specific requirements of that section before dismissing it because another section has a greater claim. Let each department put its case and listen carefully to all of the others.

The role of the practice manager is one of support for each of the partners who are acting as heads of department. The duties delegated to the practice manager will be directly proportional to the ability of the partners to delegate and to the ability of the practice manager to accomplish the task. The way forward is greater delegation by partners and greater accomplishment by the manager.

Chapter 15

Retirement

John Gripper

Age of retirement

Many veterinary surgeons in practice used to work long after the normally accepted retirement age because they had made insufficient provision for their own private pension and could not afford to live off the state retirement pension.

Times have changed – veterinary surgeons in government and commercial appointments often have a compulsory retirement age of 60. There is a growing tendency for those in general practice to retire at 60 or even in their mid 50s. This has been influenced by the increase in property prices over the years combined with the reduction from 60 to 50 as the age when Capital Gains Tax retirement relief can be claimed.

After 25 or 30 years, practice can lose its challenge and many veterinary surgeons look to develop their hobbies or outside interests for mental stimulation. One advantage of an earlier retirement age is that it provides an opportunity to pursue a second career on a part time basis such as a consultant or adviser. Work can be undertaken on a voluntary basis for animal charities at home or overseas, or to set up a totally new business venture.

Planning for retirement

An attempt must be made to calculate and predict your likely income and expenditure after you have retired. Mortgage and children's education should have been completed and pension premium payments stopped or reduced. Most pension policies are planned to mature between ages 60 to 70 but will provide a lower pension if taken earlier.

If your likely income is not going to be sufficient then plans should be made for you or your spouse to look for an alternative source of income. Reductions of expenditure may have to be made such as only running one car between you.

For those who have left practice some expenditure that has been taken for granted such as phone bills, postage stamps, stationery and even little items in the office such as paperclips can come as a bit of a shock when you have to pay for them out of your own pocket.

Some practitioners are reluctant to 'cut the cord' with their old practice and would like to continue working on a part-time basis. Subject to an agreement of the continuing partners or the purchaser of the practice to continue to work on a mutually agreed basis, this may be useful for a short time, especially if the retiring partner has some special veterinary expertise, but it is not always a happy arrangement in the long term.

New ideas and changes will take place in the practice and it is not always helpful to have the old boss still hanging around while these changes come about. Often the best advice is to make a clean break from your old practice and look for pastures new.

Where to live

A major decision has to made about where to live after your retirement. Do you stay put where your friends are, move to a part of the country to be nearer to your grandchildren, or buy a bungalow on the south coast?

Be very wary of moving abroad. That lovely summer villa where you drink wine by the poolside with your friends can turn into a lonely place in the cold wet winter and the Spanish hospitals are not the place to be treated for pneumonia or have that prostate operation.

If you are going to have a shortage of income it may be sensible to cash in on your property assets by selling your house and moving to a smaller house in an area where property values are cheaper – the capital saved from the move can be invested to provide a useful income or used to purchase an annuity. The smaller house will have lower running expenses.

When deciding where you plan to live in your retirement do think ahead to when you will be older and infirm and may not even be able to drive. Are the local shops within easy walking distance? Do you really want a large garden that needs the lawn cut each week? The weeding can become a burden to you when you are crippled with arthritis and cannot afford a gardener.

Sale of practice or partnership

Your deed of partnership should set out the arrangements for the valuation and sale of the practice assets. Sometimes the deed will have been written many years ago and not been updated. This can lead to problems if the method of goodwill valuation is either outdated or not specified.

Difficulties can also arise over the method of valuation of property and the instructions given to the valuer. 'Open market value' as between willing buyer and seller is the usual method for residential property. However for practice premises it may be necessary to value on the basis of 'continuing veterinary use' or even current building costs in the case of a purpose built veterinary hospital. If the site has a potential development value that may have to be taken into account in the property valuation.

Subject to your age and Capital Gains Tax position you are probably advised to take your practice capital assets in cash rather than having an income over the years which would be subject to income tax. Capital can always produce income (often tax free) but it is far harder to turn income into capital. However there are some tax advantages for both you and your spouse if each retain a small source of earned income. If you can run a small business or 'consultancy' from your home then you can offset some of your costs against tax, i.e. motor expenses, telephone, use of office at home, postage stamps and even buy those paperclips through the business.

However it may be that the practice property is more valuable than is needed for the incoming purchaser and that you can only complete a sale of the rest of the practice by retaining ownership of the practice property, leasing it to the buyer with an option to purchase at a later date.

If you decide to sell your practice it is important that you have a professional valuation of the property, goodwill and other assets before you put it onto the market, and try to maintain the maximum degree of confidentiality until the sale has been completed.

Capital Gains Tax

You will be liable to pay Capital Gains Tax (CGT) on the sale of your goodwill and practice property. Your own private residence is exempt but if this has been used for business purposes there may a liability for CGT on the business proportion of your private house.

The rules are that if part of your private house has been used *solely for business purposes* then a proportional part of the gain will be liable for CGT. However no tax is payable if one or more rooms *are only partly used for business purposes*, even if some of the running costs of the house have been claimed against profits for income tax purposes.

The Finance Act 1998 introduced fundamental changes to the structure of CGT. The old retirement relief with indexation is to be phased out over 5 years up to 5 April 2003. From 5 April 1998 there will be the introduction of a taper relief with different rates applicable to business assets and non-business assets.

There is a personal exemption from CGT in that an individual will not be charged on the first £7100 (1999/2000) of taxable gain in one year. Capital losses can be used to offset against gains in the same year but not rolled forward.

The partner or principal must be over the age of 50 (or earlier if you suffer from ill health) and the scale for both retirement relief and taper relief will be reduced on a sliding scale if the asset has been held for less than ten years. In the interim period up to 2003, a combination of both retirement and taper relief will be available.

In order to claim the business relief you must still be the owner or part owner of the business. For example if you sell your practice but retain ownership of the practice property which you rent out to the new practice then this property becomes an investment asset and not a business and will not be eligible for full business retirement relief on a sale at a later date.

Rollover reliefs are also available when the proceeds from the sale of your business can be reinvested into a new business or venture capital fund one year before or three years after the disposal of your business asset.

The new business need not be related to the old business, for example you could sell a veterinary practice and buy a book shop. The advantage of rollover relief is that it postpones the CGT until you sell the second asset, at which time you can once again roll over your gain or claim retirement relief.

Sickness and health

Retirement is an ideal time to get fit. Have a medical check up and a good hard look at your body in front of a mirror. You have a third of your life left to live so it is important to be positive and lead an active life both physically and mentally in your retirement or you will just degenerate.

If you are overweight, go on a controlled diet. Start regular exercise: join a fitness class or a gym, go swimming or cycling, take up tennis, squash or golf, go jogging or hiking and lose that double chin and excess weight around the middle.

If you are having to retire because of ill health remember that it is possible to claim benefits from the state up to the age of 65, whether you have been employed or self-employed. From 6 April 1995, a new State Incapacity Benefit replaced sickness and invalidity benefits. There is an objective medical test for incapacity over 28 weeks, also the earnings-related element is abolished, and the benefit is taxable.

State retirement pension

At age 65 for men and 60 for women there is an entitlement to the state retirement pension. Married women have to wait until their husband reaches the age of 65 unless they are entitled to a pension in their own right.

This pension need not be collected each week from the post office but a monthly transfer of money can be made to your bank account.

If you are still earning after the age of 65 and paying income tax at the higher rate then it may be tax advantageous to postpone taking the state retirement pension. When you decide to postpone your pension you will receive a pension enhanced by $7^{1}/_{2}$p a week for each £1 for each year of postponed retirement after the age of 65. However you cannot postpone the pension for more than five years but by the age of 70 you will have increased the payments by 37.5% for the rest of your life.

If you are entitled to any graduated retirement benefit (based on any graduated contributions you paid between 1961 and 1975) or additional pension (in respect of your earnings from April 1978) this can also be postponed and increased by $7\frac{1}{2}\%$ each year until age 70.

Once you reach the pension age of 65 for men and 60 for women there is no need for you to pay any further National Insurance contributions, but your employer's share will have to be paid at the 'not contracted' rate.

Retirement annuities and personal pensions

Despite the virtue of putting aside funds each year to pay premiums for adequate personal pensions, sadly there are still some veterinary surgeons who have not paid enough into their retirement pension schemes.

All is not lost if you are still earning a self employed income after your retirement from practice, then you can continue with your tax free premiums each year. The individual tax relief for annual premiums for personal pensions paid over the age of 61 are 40% of net relevant earnings. If you are still earning after your retirement then you can continue with your tax free premiums each year.

The annual premiums that can be paid over the age of 61 are 40% of net relevant earnings for personal pensions and 27% of net relevant earnings for retirement annuities.

Drawing your pension

Careful planning is needed in deciding when to cash in your pension policies. If you have no immediate need of the pension money then you can elect to have your policies 'paid up' and with both the with profit policies and the unit linked funds they will continue to grow and benefit from the annual bonus or increase in the value of the units. Payout on death can either be a return of fund or return of premiums plus interest.

This is of particular importance to the terminal bonus which can represent a large part of the final payment. This terminal bonus is affected by the strength of the investment success achieved by the insurance company over the years and the number of years that your policy has been in existence.

When you decide to cash in on your pension annuity the first decision is whether to take the maximum cash free sum or opt for a larger pension. For personal pensions the maximum cash free sum is 25% of the fund whilst for the older style retirement annuities it is $33\frac{1}{3}\%$.

The value of your fund will purchase an annuity and you should not just accept the offer made by your insurance company. Take advantage of the 'open market option' which allows you (or your insurance broker) to research the market and obtain the best annuity rates from any insurance company. There is a surprising difference in the annuity rates on offer and you must use the open market option to get the best rates.

Annuity rates are influenced by your age, sex and the level of current interest rates. It would therefore pay to delay cashing in your pension when annuity rates are low. Other choices are as to whether to take out a joint annuity with your spouse at a reduced amount which continues to pay a pension at a lower rate to your spouse after your death. This decision will depend on you and your own financial circumstances.

There is also an option to take out an escalating pension that will increase by a set percentage each year (3% or 5%) or even can be fully index linked to RPI. The payments for the first few years will be much lower but if you think that you or your spouse are likely to live to 80+ then it could be a shrewd move.

Another option available is a unit linked pension which is directly linked to the performance of the stock market through a unit trust. Here you will find that the initial pension payments will be lower than the traditional annuity but could rise depending on the success of your investment performance.

There are some advantages if you have a number of pension policies with different companies as this allows you more flexibility in that you can continue to pay premiums into some policies but make the others 'paid up'. The 'paid up' policies can be transferred to other existing policies if you wish but there may be a small cost involved.

At a later date you can cash in the policies as you need the extra income but choosing the best time to obtain good annuity rates. You can also select and vary the types of annuities you elect to receive.

New flexible annuities have been introduced that will allow you to take out the tax free sum, draw some annuity but postpone the main annuity payments.

Income drawdown allows you to take an income and the tax-free lump sum from your pension fund, without the need to take an annuity up until the age of 75 years. However look carefully at the amount of commissions that you will pay for these income drawdown schemes.

Investments

You will probably have some capital to invest from the sale of your practice, maturing endowment and life policies and the cash sum from your pension annuities.

Decide first if you wish to invest this capital in the stock market directly into shares of your choice or through unit trusts and investment trusts. Do you want an investment that produces income or capital growth or a mixture of the two? You also need to decide the element of risk you wish to take.

Then take advice from a reputable stockbroker to put together a suitable portfolio which is tailor-made to fit your needs of bonds and equities. £7000 a year can go into an ISA which is free of both income tax and capital gains tax.

Do not be seduced into any 'get rich quick' schemes like high interest gilt edged stock in Gibraltar, traded options, dubious venture capital schemes, ostrich farming, enticing share offers with an Amsterdam or Indonesian postmark, loans to Nigerian businessmen, or a Lloyds syndicate specialising in asbestosis reinsurance.

Inheritance tax

List all your assets and put a value on them. The time of retirement is an opportunity to take a careful look into the future and decide if you can pass on some capital to your children. It is often more helpful for them to have capital when they are struggling with high mortgage payments and school fees than later on in life when they are financially self-sufficient.

In 2000/01 the first £234 000 of your estate on death has a nil rate band. Thereafter the remainder is subject to a 40% tax. No inheritance tax is paid on transfers between husband and wife.

Each year annual gifts can be made per donor of £3000 without tax. Gifts made out of income and small gifts of up to £250 per donee are also exempt, as are gifts up to £5000 by a parent to a bride or groom. No inheritance tax is payable on lifetime gifts between individuals provided that the gift is made seven years before the death. There is a tapering relief for gifts made between three and seven years before death.

Have a look at your will to make sure that it is written to take full advantage of the tax legislation. Assets should be divided between spouses to ensure that both estates can claim the £234 000 nil rate band and if possible this sum should be left directly to the family on the first death.

It is possible to gift your house to the family but you will have to pay a market rent and the family will be responsible for the repairs. You will then have to live for seven years to get the full inheritance tax benefit. Gifts to charities are free of inheritance tax whether made during life or on death. Insurance policies can be taken out to pay the likely inheritance tax or you can set up a trust.

Even if your will does not take into account the latest legislation all is not lost because it is possible for your beneficiaries to rewrite your will under a Deed of Variation. This has to take place within two years of death, subject to unanimous agreement by all the beneficiaries and can be rewritten to take full tax advantage of the distribution of monies from your estate.

Summary

Retirement should be carefully thought through and sensible plans made for the future. It is a time of challenge for what lies ahead, not dis-appointment at what might have been. As you shut one door, another will open and it is up to each individual to ensure that this new door will lead to a productive, satisfying and enjoyable way of life.

Chapter 16
The Practice Manager
John Bower

The university veterinary course trains us all to be competent diagnosticians, physicians and surgeons. It does not, as yet, take into account that as practitioners we have to be able to run a business. In short, we are trained to be assistant veterinary surgeons and are expected to glean information on all aspects of practice finance and management during our first few years in practice. However, most final year veterinary students now attend the innovative BVA/SPVS First Postgraduate Job Symposium which takes place immediately prior to the start of their final year. This is entirely devoted to the non-clinical aspects of general practice and to some extent corrects this omission in the veterinary course.

In order to carry out efficient management of his practice, a veterinary surgeon must either spend time on it after working hours at the family's expense or during the normal working day with the loss of clinical time.

A practice manager can fill a role in the practice that makes the practice more productive and problem free. He or she should take on the more mundane tasks in running a practice, giving the practitioner more time to do the thing he does best – practising veterinary medicine and surgery. Possibly even more importantly, he gives the practitioner time to think. In my experience, the leaps and bounds in practice expansion have come when I have taken the time to just sit and think about where the practice is going. This important aspect of practice management should not be overlooked.

The practice secretary is indeed a type of manager and performs many non-clinical tasks in the practice. In many practices a partner or principal may enjoy the role of manager. There are, however, specific areas in the practice where the non-veterinary manager can relieve us of those tasks that we are either all performing without realising it or more frequently ignoring, to the detriment of the practice.

Reception and waiting room

The nurses or receptionists have to be trained, not just thrown in at the deep end. They must be told or shown how to handle people, both face to face and on the telephone. Neglect in this area will have disastrous effects on practice growth. The practice manager takes on the role or delegates it to senior reception staff, but then monitors progress and corrects any problems.

He is responsible for the patient records, their computerisation or filing, and storage. He orders further supplies when needed. He works out the appointment system if applicable and is highly involved in the method of fee payment. It is the manager, not the veterinary surgeon, who monitors and corrects this and devises the method by which the practice cashes up and balances the till. An important area of his responsibility is the setting up or maintaining of an efficient vaccine booster reminder system – and then ensuring the system is adhered to by receptionists, nurses and veterinary surgeons alike. In a busy practice this simple task, if efficiently and diligently performed may pay his entire salary. If in doubt, work out what difference an extra two or three vaccination boosters (i.e. consultations) per day would make to the annual turnover.

During computerisation, and this is the way practice systems must surely go in the future, with many practices already computerised, someone has to set up the computer. A practice manager can devote time to this and will ensure other staff members are familiar with the methodology.

In general the practice manager keeps a tight rein on all the practice reception area activities. And he is available to discuss clients' financial queries – a situation in which a third party is often at an advantage.

Practice office

The practice office is the hub of the practice and it is here that the practice manager performs his most time consuming and valuable role – that of problem solving. This includes staff problems, equipment breakdown, premises or car repair, financial problems and clients' financial queries and complaints. These problems crop up regularly, when least expected and needed, and certainly more than one at a time. A perfectly acceptable day's clinical work can be ruined by a difficult staff problem or malfunctioning autoclave, and a practice manager is worth employing for this aspect alone. Staff problems become easier because the practice manager automatically attracts the first approach. Both veterinary surgeon and nurse rotas are his responsibility and any variations are requested through him. Pay negotiations and holiday requests are initiated through him also. It is his responsibility to ensure that enough staff are available at any one time to perform the various duties within the practice. These tasks should be undertaken by discussion with the veterinarians and nurses, and the reduction in stress for the principal or partners by delegation of the task is considerable.

The responsibility of hiring (and in some circumstances firing) can be given to him. For certain categories of staff this can be his complete responsibility but if preferred it can be under partners' supervision. We find this aspect particularly helpful and time-saving in the initial advertising for, and interviewing of, reception staff, student nurses and office staff. The partners are then involved only in interviewing those shortlisted and have none of the hassle of the early stages.

A worthwhile exercise is to draw up a job description for each member of the practice including the manager. The employee should draw up his own and then the partner or principal, or practice manager should set down what they see as the role and by comparing the two efforts, a final version can be agreed. An occasional review by the manager of personnel roles on a one to one basis is of benefit and should include a two way discussion as to how each employee is fulfilling his role, and how practical and accurate is the job description (see also Chapter 12).

Finance

Practice finance is of course his forte. The administration of VAT, wage calculations, payments and even negotiations become a thing of the past for the partners. He can deal with these entirely and make recommendations to the partners for a final decision. A close watch on practice profitability should be kept by him with appropriate advice on pricing and fee structure to achieve the desired profitability. Professional fees should be reviewed at least annually and with computerisation can be adjusted by small percentages as often as needed. Drug prices should be reviewed on receipt of each invoice and are updated automatically on computers by veterinary wholesalers and computer companies. The practice manager should be involved in formulating and supervising the systems for collecting cash within the practice and should minimise the bad debt level. One's staff are better at collecting bad debts than outside agencies and the practice manager should be able to help in this area – at the very least by telephone calls to clients whose accounts are long overdue.

Budgeting is an essential part of practice management. The practice manager should prepare a budget annually and present it to the partners some three months before the start of the next financial year.

To enable sensible business decisions to be taken, it is necessary to know exactly how the practice is faring at any given moment. To this end we have a monthly evening meeting involving the five partners and the manager. The venue is away from the practice to ensure there are no interruptions. At this meeting our manager presents us with a profit and loss account relating to the previous month and the year so far, compares our performance against budget, and talks through the various headings. Thus we know if takings are up or down, if expenses are outstripping income, and in effect how profitable the practice is on a monthly basis. The end of year accounts are history, so these monthly accounts enable us to make minor adjustments when they are needed to prevent disastrous years or to ensure an adequate surplus. In addition we are able to discuss and solve personnel and other problems that occur from time to time in the practice. We require the manager to discuss in depth any deviations from budget. He must explain it and outline ways to correct it to ensure budget profit for the year is delivered.

He can help in the marketing of veterinary services by collating information for, and arranging the printing of, practice newsletters, by organising client meetings and open days, ensuring entries in *Yellow Pages* are up to date, or, for instance, setting up obesity or geriatric clinics. The possibilities are endless; the common factor is that he generates original ideas or takes on board those of partners, assistants or nurses and then progresses them. The only limiting factors are his brief and his enthusiasm.

The maintenance and upkeep of practice premises become his responsibility so that a partner no longer needs to be concerned if a pipe is leaking or redecoration is needed. Even the organisation of the cleaning of the practice becomes his responsibility in conjunction with other staff.

Personnel management

In a practice of any size, personnel management is important, and in larger practices this can occupy a large part of the practice manager's time. Some practices these days are so large that they employ a full time personnel manager, which shows that interpersonal relationships are all important in team building. When you consider that relationships between members of the team, and working conditions are so high up in the list of motivators, this aspect of the practice manager's work should not be neglected. Periodic appraisals are an important part of this and are dealt with fully in Chapter 12.

Disadvantages

There are of course potential disadvantages to having a practice manager, the first of which is cost. As the position is one of responsibility, his wage should be roughly on a par with an assistant veterinary surgeon. Initially it may not be necessary to employ a manager full time, thus enabling an assessment of his value to be made economically.

Loss of familiarity with routine financial affairs by the partners rapidly ensues and can be regarded as a disadvantage.

For years the principal or partner will have been the one to deal with fee complaints, account queries, etc. Clients may not take kindly to the new arrangement which may insulate the principal from them. The amount of responsibility delegated in this field will vary from practice to practice.

Diversion of personnel problems away from a partner can also lead to a loss of awareness of what is going on in the practice. It is easy to take less interest in the general running of the practice with consequent loss of dynamism and sometimes profitability.

If you resent delegating responsibilities to an employee and wish to retain total control, a practice manager is not for you because one of the great advantages is that, while he frees you of the mundane tasks involved in running the practice, you obviously retain ultimate control. Any major decision has to be approved by the partners before being executed.

Qualities required

The qualities needed in a practice manager depend on the area of responsibility he or she is to be given. If this is to be mainly finance and staff administration, then an accountancy background may be advisable, but as many tasks within the practice are easier with a knowledge of problems likely to be encountered, drug names and veterinary systems, a veterinary nurse with an interest in this area may be ideal. A person with medical hospital administration experience should be considered, as should a retired services person with secretarial and management training. The main qualities required are an organised mind and the ability to get on with people and integrate into the practice. He or she must be capable of being assertive and able to deal with people tactfully, and preferably should choose the position as a career not just as a job. Because the practice manager absorbs all the stress that drops from the shoulders of the practice owner, he must be able to take a certain amount himself.

In a single handed practice, the manager is often the veterinary surgeon's spouse. This works well in these circumstances but in my opinion only in these circumstances. In a larger practice, the employment of a spouse with responsibility, assumed or otherwise, over other staff members can greatly increase the stress and decrease the morale of a practice and must be handled very carefully indeed. I have seen it work only very rarely and all too often it can cause severe problems.

The size of the practice to some extent governs the need for a manager. I first employed a practice manager in 1973 when the practice consisted of a principal, two assistants and three nurses. He was a retired naval officer, who had no problems with accepting his role in the practice. He started as a part time employee but his work rapidly expanded until he was needed full time. He enabled me to spend far more time on clinical work and continuing professional development, more time with clients and more time in thinking about the direction the practice should be taking. The importance of all four to the practice future should not be underestimated. The practice now has 10 veterinarians with some 30 support staff so the decision would seem to have been justified. In addition stress was reduced considerably. It is difficult to concentrate on unusual medical cases and complicated surgical procedures if a major staff problem is weighing heavily on one's mind. Stress leads to lack of concentration which leads to mistakes. The freedom created by leaving problem solving to someone else while still retaining the control and direction of the practice makes the employment of a practice manager well worth considering for this reason alone.

The future

From small beginnings in veterinary practice, as our profession has developed, so has the role of practice management. The need for efficient management of the practice is now fully accepted, and the number of practice managers in regular employment, whether veterinarians or otherwise, is now rapidly increasing. Two national associations exist for the development of management ideas – the Society of Practising Veterinary Surgeons (SPVS) and the Veterinary Practice Management Association (VPMA). Both are involved in practice management but SPVS have been for many years also involved in other aspects of general practice for veterinary surgeons. The VPMA was formed in 1991 in response to the specific needs of the practice manager (both veterinary and non-veterinary), and now has around 500 members. Both associations hold an annual meeting and frequent seminars for the exchange of ideas.

The VPMA, adapting a format used by the Veterinary Hospital Managers Association in the USA, developed a qualification for practice managers in 1996 – the Certificate in Veterinary Practice Management (CVPM). These certificates are awarded by examination, usually in the spring of each year, and are of a very high standrd. Quite a number of managers and veterinary surgeons have now gained this qualification and have brought added skills to their practices. There is no doubt that this aspect of veterinary practice will develop, and that it will be to the benefit of our profession. The CVPM will surely be a prerequisite in the future for the practice manager.

It was recognised though, that as this is a 'gold standard' qualification, it was not possible for someone inexperienced in practice management to contemplate enrolling for it until they had been involved for some time. Thus an entry-level qualification was needed. The Education Committee of the VPMA has now developed such a qualification, the Veterinary Practice Administration Certificate (VPAC). This will be run in colleges throughout the country in conjunction with the Open College Network, and is already proving popular with people wishing to become involved in the management side of veterinary practice.

Chapter 17
The Practice Manual
John Bower

A problem that occurs in all but the smallest practice is that of communication between the staff – the team members. This problem increases as the practice grows and even the basic practice rules and policies can fail to reach everyone. Regular practice meetings, practice bulletins, memos and word of mouth all have their place, but a 'practice manual' is an extremely useful vehicle for drawing it all together.

The concept is that of a working manual, applicable to one's own practice, containing subjects of interest and use to all. It becomes the standard reference for such diverse subjects as history of the practice, aims and objectives, standards of dress, holiday policy, grievance procedures, meetings schedules, telephone usage, policy on smoking, etc. We have a section on COSHH Regulations, and health and safety as they apply to our practice – large sections indeed but an essential reference for each employee.

A suggested layout for the various sections and contents is shown below.

Contents

By way of illustration, I have picked out at random some sections of our own practice manual. I have included a job description, sections on practice hours, absence through sickness, dress and demeanour, behaviour, and professional negligence.

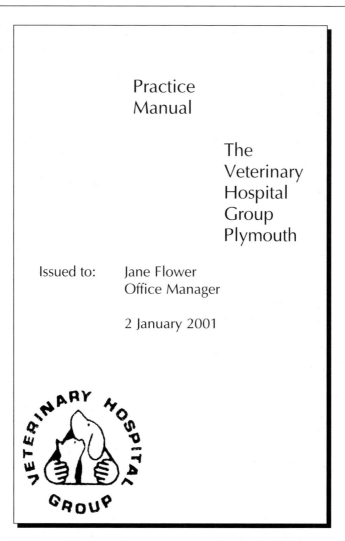

Figure 17.1 A practice manual ensures everyone knows the basic practice rules and policies.

A.3 Job description

Job Title: **Office manager**
Responsible to: Practice manager
Responsible for: Practice secretary

Duties

General duties: The office manager is responsible for:

- Ensuring that the office is kept tidy and well organised, and runs smoothly.
- Updating systems and procedures as necessary, working with the practice manager.
- Coordinating marketing reports and mailshots using the veterinary software, in association with other departments.

Daily responsibilities include:

- Coordinating the daily workload for the practice secretary.
- Processing the daily takings of the veterinary hospital which involves reconciling the figures, payment of monies to the bank and running daily transaction report.

Weekly responsibilities include:

- Updating spreadsheets using information received from various sources for all surgeries.
- Attending heads of departments meetings.

Monthly responsibilities include:

- Processing payment of invoices by cheque and completing all necessary paper/computer work following the cheque run.
- Reconciling receipts and payments to the bank statement.
- Compiling profit and loss account for the group.
- Generating reminders for vaccinations, producing letters to clients and analysing data to find out success rate of the reminders.
- Credit control, working with the head receptionist.

3.4 Practice hours

Normal working hours are 09.00 to 18.30 with one hour for lunch. Many staff work a longer day and this is appreciated by partners and clients alike. Good time keeping is of considerable importance and a matter of courtesy to the clients who expect us to be available.

Nights and weekends on duty are necessary and scheduled to fit in with the practice rota.

Time keeping. We do not expect anyone to clock in or out of work. Your normal weekly rota expectations will be quoted in your contract or letter of appointment. We do expect you to familiarise yourself with your rota which is posted several weeks in advance, and we expect prompt time keeping at the beginning of each period of working. Where telephone answering is involved this is particularly important. Where lateness was unavoidable we expect time to be made up without recompense. The nature of the work we do demands that, on occasions, it is necessary to do emergency work outside the normal hours of work, and finishing times have to be varied.

Consistent poor time keeping will not be tolerated and may lead to a formal warning and/or dismissal in extreme instances.

3.6 Absence through sickness

(a) It is the responsibility of *all* practice members absent through sickness or injury to inform the practice manager by 08.30 on the first day of absence. Thereafter you must keep the practice manager informed as to your condition and your anticipated date for returning to work. Other members of staff receiving the above information first are to pass this on to the practice manager.

(b) Please note that there is no statutory legislation that requires the practice to pay an employee until Statutory Sick Pay starts after three continuous days of sickness.

(c) If absent more than three consecutive working days, a certificate signed by a registered medical practitioner is to be sent to the head of your department as soon as is practicable, and in any case within 72 hours. In this connection, the practice will accept the certificate supplied by the medical practitioner for the use of the Department of Health. If necessary the practice manager will forward the certificate to the employee's local office of the DSS. Where your doctor makes a charge for this, the practice will reimburse you on receipt of an invoice.

(d) Maternity leave: government legislation sets out detailed conditions which the employer and expectant mother must meet for maternity leave. If you are pregnant you should ask the practice to provide you with the current information at the time in question. We comply with statutory requirements for maternity leave.

Continues

3.6 Absence through sickness *continued*

(e) Pregnancy: you should let the practice know as soon as your pregnancy is confirmed so that we can ensure you avoid any unnecessary risks to you or your baby. These could include X-rays, handling some animal tissues or waste products, or certain drugs. It is most important that you wash your hands frequently using the disinfectant provided. In addition read the sections relating to X-radiation in this manual and notices posted in the X-ray rooms.

(f) All absences will be recorded and detailed to any future employer for reference purposes.

3.9 Dress and demeanour

You should dress appropriately to the post you hold. People working at the reception desk are the public face of the practice and create the first impression to a client. The standard of dress you adopted for your interview should be reflected in the way you dress for work daily. First impressions are easily created and are very difficult to change once established. Your appearance, dress and attitude all influence the first impression.

The appearance of all staff is considered by the partners to be extremely important in terms of meeting with our client's expectations. Staff are expected to appear neat, clean and tidy with appropriate dress as detailed below. All staff members are identified by name badges or embroidered uniform.

Veterinary nurses:

- Bottle Green VN uniform. Tunic, Trousers or Dress of appropriate size, design and length. All fastenings should be intact and the uniform ironed.
- Bottle Green Belt and Buckle issued with dress.
- Black tights, stockings or socks with appropriate uniform.
- Sensible, comfortable, flat, enclosed black shoes. In summer enclosed sandals may be worn, coloured black, white or tan. Boots, flip-flops and other forms of footwear are not acceptable.
- Bottle Green VH Waistcoats.
- Bottle Green Sweatshirts.
- VN badge on the collar.

Student veterinary nurses:

- Green/White striped uniform. Tunic, Bottle Green Trousers or Dress of appropriate size, design and length. All fastenings should be intact and the uniform ironed.

Continued

3.9 Dress and demeanour *continued*

- Belt (black for year 1, grey for year 2) and buckle issued with dress.
- Black tights, stockings or socks with appropriate uniform.
- Sensible, comfortable, flat, enclosed black shoes. In summer enclosed sandals may be worn, coloured black, white or tan. Boots, flip-flops and other forms of footwear are not acceptable.
- Bottle Green VH Waistcoats.
- Bottle Green Sweatshirts.

3.10 Behaviour

Any behaviour which reflects badly on the practice or profession should be avoided. In particular you should avoid giving offence to a client or potential client. Dealing with an angry or aggressive client can be difficult and you should ask a senior member of the practice or a partner for help. You should never argue with, or be rude or offensive to a client. Rather refer them to a partner, veterinarian, or the practice manager in the knowledge that if you have carried out your task to the best of your ability, we will always back you up. Refer to the *Practice Resource Manual* (published by BSAVA) for particular help with types of problems.

Some specific aspects of personal behaviour need particular mention. The illegal use of prohibited substances at any time, but specifically on practice premises, is incompatible with employment in this practice. The presence on our premises of dangerous and controlled drugs makes this provision mandatory. If such misuse is discovered or suspected, you may be dismissed without further warning. **This document is formal warning of our policy.**

4.2 Professional negligence

Any person who becomes aware of circumstances giving rise to any possibility, however remote, that a claim for negligence might be made against the practice must immediately give notice thereof to the partners with written details of the facts and circumstances.

Under no circumstances are you to admit liability to a client for anything that goes wrong with a case. This would immediately nullify our Professional Indemnity. Of course sympathy must be extended to the client; this is not an admission of negligence.

The practice manual is issued to each employee as they join the practice, and is personalised to include their job description. Each employee signs for the receipt of the manual, and by so doing, agrees to abide by the code of conduct it contains. The reaction to the manual is generally that it is very useful, especially for new team members to understand the practice ethics more quickly, but it is also a valuable reminder for long term staff. It is, of course, constantly subject to updating, and as it is produced in a looseleaf binding, or stapled form, this is easy to achieve. Once the basic manual has been produced on the practice computer, it is a simple matter to amend, update and print new or additional copies.

Having seen our own practice grow through all stages from single-handed to 10 veterinarians, I contend that a practice manual is essential for an efficiently managed large practice. In retrospect, however, I would certainly have found it useful much earlier, even at the three vet stage at which I first employed a practice manager.

Chapter 18
Business Marketing

Peter Gripper

Over the last decade the value of marketing has been appreciated by many veterinary businesses and has resulted in many practices improving their profits by embracing the marketing ethos, developing services and expanding their business.

The Institute of Marketing defines marketing as 'The process which identifies, anticipates and supplies customer requirements efficiently and profitably' and it is the emphasis on customer needs that is essential to this process.

The real difference between selling and marketing is that marketing considers the needs of the customer, whereas selling considers the needs of the vendor. It is worth noting that if the customer's needs are met then the vendor's needs, by way of increased profit, will also be met.

Within this chapter I have used the word 'products', in a broad sense and it refers to the service and services that are offered by a particular practice or individual and not just to 'medicines'.

The practices that have accepted and embraced the philosophy of marketing realise that the emphasis is primarily on the customer's needs and secondly that the process involves the whole practice. You must decide your aims, set realistic targets and get all staff to provide input to the marketing process so that the end result is a common approach, that has support throughout the business and to which staff are committed.

Stages of the marketing process

External audit

The first step is to carry out an external audit and look at external factors that can and will influence the business. Not all of these can be predicted and many are outside your control, but a simple example would be to look at local employment prospects. If half of the town is employed by a single large national company that has just announced 2000 job redundancies over the next two years then the local economy is likely to be in decline.

Factors to be considered include political issues, environmental issues, the economy, social, technological and legislative issues. For example the political influences and debate regarding dog ownership or farm subsidies will have an influence. The environmental impact of clinical and pharmaceutical waste disposal is relevant as is any associated legislation that accompanies it. The national economic climate and the local economic climate may be entirely different. Technological advances have resulted in many practices installing their own laboratory facility and imaging suites, with scanners for cardio work, as well as reproductive ultrasound and embryo transfer work in cattle practices. These and many other issues need careful consideration and anticipation of how current changes are going to affect the business.

Internal audit

The next stage of the marketing process is an internal audit. Too many decisions are based on assumptions about what is happening and too often people's gut feeling is the basis for decision when quantitative data is to hand. The internal audit allows you a far better understanding of what contributes to the success of your business and it looks at far more than just financial aspects. The internal audit will establish what is currently happening in the business and produce information that can be used for future decision making.

Data collected in this audit may include, for example,

- how many clients you have
- how often you see your clients
- what their average spend is with you at each occasion
- what percentage of work is operations
- what percentage of work is vaccinations
- what percentage of work is neutering
- how much work is second opinion work.

On the large animal side similar information is needed regarding

- how many cows each farm has
- how many youngstock on each farm
- what is the average spend per cow per year
- what percentage of turnover is service income
- what percentage of turnover is drug income.

Upon completion of the audit you will have a much better idea of your business and what its constituent parts are.

Pareto's Law (better known as the 80:20 rule) states that 80% of your work is derived from 20% of your clients. It is still valid and can be extended further to other areas of the business. For example, in large animal practice 80% of medicine income may be derived from 20% of the product range and two groups of products, dry cow and milking cow intramammaries, may account for quite a large proportion of income. On the small animals side routine vaccination, boosters and neutering procedures can account for a large part of annual income.

Before everyone totally ignores the 20% that makes up the 'smaller' customers, it is worth noting that the best potential for growth are the customers in this 20% group.

Setting targets and planning

Armed with this information objectives can be set for the short and long term, and targets must then be determined. It is most important to set targets that are realistic, achievable and measurable.

Long term and strategic planning must work hand in hand with the short term and operational planning to achieve the common targets. This planning stage is an important part of the process and considers the four P's, *product*, *price*, *promotion* and *place*. This chapter is not intended to discuss pricing policy which is covered elsewhere in this book.

In many instances individual customer requirements are different and although several groups or types may be apparent this has to be catered for in the plan. From the internal audit you will have a good profile of your customers and you need to know your customers if you are going to meet their needs.

Once completed, the marketing plan has to be published and everyone should be a part of it. In the early planning stages everyone should have had a chance to comment. The final plan therefore includes input from all the staff in the business and so everyone has the same objectives and the same strategies to achieve them. It is far more likely that targets will be achieved if everyone has contributed to the plan.

The final part of the planning process is to monitor the progress of the plan, and to revise it accordingly when there are changes in circumstances. The market place is ever changing; new customers may appear, more or less direct competition may arise, new products and technological developments will alter the situation and so constant revision is necessary.

Using the marketing plan

Reviewing the marketing plan is the end of the process and also the start. When completed it has taken you full circle because new objectives will have been set and new strategies determined to achieve them.

When reviewing the marketing plan consider how your own situation differs from 'perfect competition'. With perfect competition there are

❑ many suppliers, and no one dominates
❑ many purchasers, who are unable individually to exert pressure on suppliers
❑ one supplier's products are the same as others
❑ there is free entry into the market
❑ 'perfect knowledge' is assumed. i.e. everyone knows what is being offered and at what price.

To be successful one should aim to have a competitive differential advantage which can be obtained in any or all of the areas above. Offering better products (services, drug or price) is one area on which you may decide to concentrate. Where there is not free entry into the market, for example the prescription only medicine (POM) market some practices, particularly large animal practices, may have become over reliant in this area and left themselves vulnerable if the market changes. How would a change in legislation affect practices if large animal POMs could be bought easily elsewhere? How would small animal practices be affected if vaccines were only necessary every two years or perhaps be shown to provide lifelong immunity?

Market research

Market research will illustrate how little your customer knows about your business and the products on offer. Improving knowledge to the customer is one area in which veterinary surgeons are notoriously poor. Although practices pride themselves on their knowledge, commitment and compassion, our surgical techniques and skills are still judged by the quality of our suturing.

Market research can be carried out face to face, by telephone or by post and each method has its merits and failings. You can conduct a small survey yourself in a rudimentary way by asking a few friends or current customers if they know what services the business offers – you may be very disappointed at how little they know. The best approach is to delegate to those professionally trained at market research. They will then ensure that unbiased questions are asked and that results are interpreted correctly.

Advertising

Advertising is seen as a way to increase business and it can do so. Advertising can be 'corporate' i.e. promoting the name and can be achieved in many ways, such as:

- placing advertisements directly in the local papers and journals
- sponsoring local events
- newsletters
- brochures
- speaking locally at schools
- speaking at societies and functions
- writing for local journals
- chat shows on the local radio station
- joining local associations
- becoming involved in the community that you serve.

Advertising can also be used to promote individual products by in-house seminars, workshops, direct mailings or organising client meetings.

Customer analyses

Not all customers have the same needs and one can group customers in several ways, for example into dog owners, cat owners, dairy herds, livery stables. These groups can be further defined and one useful method is to consider your customers and relate their current level of business (market share) to the potential level of business (market growth).

The Boston matrix, shown in Fig. 18.1, was used to forecast the future potential position of a product in the market place but is equally valid for veterinary practices to analyse their customer base, particularly large animal clients. Each customer can be placed into one of the four quadrants and each area has different considerations and a different approach.

	High current High potential	Low current High potential
	High current Low potential	Low current Low potential

High

Potential business

Low

Current business

High   Low

Figure 18.1 The Boston matrix.

Where do your customers fit on the Boston matrix? The *High current/ High potential* customers are few and far between but any customers in this bracket still have some room for development.

Low current/High potential customers are the ones that need developing. This is the area of greatest potential for the business and likely to give the largest return on investment. But before you offer products to these customers the reason for the Low current business has to be established and the marketing plan for this group will be different. It is important to ensure that these customers have perfect knowledge of your business and are aware of what it has to offer.

The *High current/Low potential* group of customers should be protected. They are using all of your services to the full but you would target them if you develop or introduce new services.

The *Low current/Low potential* group of customers need checking to establish why they are low potential. This position may be due to many factors and a change in any of these factors could mean the customers move into a different group and perhaps become higher potential. Such changes may be because of an upturn in the customer's economics, technological advances e.g. a new product launch, a change in farm policy or personnel, or, a changed payment method for farmers, such as premiums penalties for quality milk production.

Analysis on a simple spreadsheet will help highlight areas where you can offer these services to customers that do not already use them. Look at

	Customers								
Farm number	**1**	**2**	**3**	**4**	**5**	**6**	**7**	**8**	**9**
Products									
Dry cow tubes	Yes	Yes	Yes	Yes	Yes	Yes	Yes	Yes	Yes
Mastitis scheme		Yes	Yes			Yes	Yes		
Fertility clinics	Yes	Yes	Yes	Yes	Yes	Yes	Yes		Yes
Foot trimming	Yes	Yes		Yes		Yes		Yes	Yes
Respiratory vaccines		Yes	Yes	Yes		Yes			
DAISY		Yes	Yes		Yes			Yes	
Nutrition advice	Yes	Yes	Yes			Yes			
Worming advice	Yes	Yes		Yes			Yes	Yes	

Figure 18.2 Spreadsheet analysis for a large animal practice.

the example in Fig. 18.2 which shows a spreadsheet for a large animal practice. The blank areas are obvious.

When planning to increase business one can consider current customers, current products, new customers and new products. Ansoff's matrix (Fig. 18.3) graphically describes the risks involved with these activities and which group you decide to target. As you move around the grid from top left to bottom right the level of risk increases.

Lower risk

Current products Current customers	New products Current customers
Current products New customers	New products New customers

Higher risk

Figure 18.3 Ansoff's matrix.

It is far easier to focus on current customers and current products before progressing to new customers and new products. The exception of course is where the market changes with technological or other developments and these new concepts have to be embraced or else the market will leave you behind. Examples in small animal practice would include specialist services such as dermatology specialists, cardiology scanning or prescription diets for pets. In large animal practice examples include mastitis advisory schemes, ultrasound scanners for bovine reproduction and embryo transfer work.

Communication

It is worth remembering that our clients buy 'benefits' from us. The particular drug in a flea spray is the feature for which we may decide to purchase and stock it but the customer is not buying this; they are buying a can of flea spray which means that their dog or cat will be rid of fleas and not scratch anymore. The non-scratching is what they buy, not the chemical formula. The customer adds '... which means that ...' onto any feature and this is what helps determine the buying choice.

It therefore is in our interest to ensure that proper communication is maintained with the customer so that they know what they are getting. When promoting products the benefits must be emphasised to the customer, not necessarily the features, and in cattle practice the cost–benefit is particularly important. Wherever possible add value to the product and avoid becoming just a supplier of goods. Advice is a good way to add value.

The veterinary profession are reticent about being compared to salespeople but, in effect, they are selling themselves to their customers through their work, treatments and behaviour. All too often communication can be at fault and this is patently obvious when a misunderstanding arises and dissatisfaction is the outcome. Communication skills are an essential part of the process, they must not be overlooked and cannot be over-emphasised.

Practice development and expansion

When assessing opportunities it is important to have quantitative data to hand and to identify those customers who are potential users of some of the services they do not currently receive. The marketing plan can be used to develop your share of the market or expand the business with customers.

Once you have assessed your customer base and their needs and have completed the internal and external audits and put the marketing plan in place, the business is then in an ideal position to meet those customer needs efficiently and profitably and thereby succeed itself.

I have discussed business planning and marketing for the business as a whole, but within the overall marketing plan for the practice there will be several smaller marketing plans for specific areas or projects. These could be in several different areas, such as:

❏ product related e.g. wormer or flea preventions or vaccinations
❏ disease related e.g. respiratory disease in calves or feline leukaemia vaccination in cats
❏ speciality related e.g. cardiology or dermatology or orthopaedic.

For each plan there will be aims and objectives set and an individual marketing plan produced. The process is the same for each one and starts with the internal and external audit, followed by setting targets and devising strategies to achieve them. The review process is the important final step.

The potential market available to veterinary practices is huge and with computer analysis of practice records it is relatively easy to quantify. What data have you assessed recently? How many clients do you have? How many dogs, cats and cattle are on your list? How many have not been to see you for two years? How many clients do you lose each year? Have they left the area or changed practice?

Understanding and analysing practice performance provides the data and knowledge and that is used to develop and plan further. Growth in the practice could have been generated from a number of sources, such as new clients, or new services to the current clients. Quantifying where growth was achieved helps with future planning. A 10% growth in turnover could be due to 10% more clients, 10% more work for the current clients, 20% more work for a dwindling number of clients, a 10% price rise, or a combination of these.

What percentage of clients have vaccinated dogs? What percentage return regularly for an annual health check and revaccinations? What percentage of your cats are vaccinated against FELV? Do you monitor disease status on your livestock units? How many of your farm clients have you tested and screened for evidence of bovine viral diarrhoea, leptospirosis or infectious bovine rhinotracheitis? Do you analyse your sales of long acting antibiotic used to treat calf pneumonia; every farmer requiring treatment dispensed is a potential case for vaccination next year and advice on housing, building ventilation and herd biosecurity. Are your clients aware that you offer these services? Have you ever surveyed your clients?

Good data allows you to assess the potential market and helps devise plans to access that market.

When implementing any particular plan it is very important that all staff members should be recommending the same advice. This includes all the veterinary surgeons and all the nursing and reception staff. Practice policy and protocol is an essential ingredient in a good marketing plan. The practice policy will determine clinical protocols that everyone in the practice can follow and recommend.

For example, the practice policy for worming adult dogs and cats might recommend worming every three months, i.e. four times a year. Your records may show that for a one vet small animal practice there are 4000 dogs and 4000 cats on the records. The potential market is therefore 16 000 doses of dog wormer per year and 16 000 doses of cat wormer each year. How many doses did you supply last year? Do your clients purchase this elsewhere or are they not aware of the clinical benefits of regular worming?

There are few markets where you can supply 100% of the market but do you currently supply 5% of this market? Could you supply 30% of the market?

Assuming that the average dog weighs 15 kg and the cost of dosing is just under £2.00 per dose then the potential market is £32 000 per year. For cats a similar calculation calculates the potential market to be £26 000 per year. For a single-handed vet practice the total market is therefore in the order of £58 000 per year.

You may be supplying 5% of the market already but if you supplied 35% of the potential market you would increase total practice turnover by over £17 000 per annum, and profit accordingly. There are many other areas that can be considered with regard to supply of products, and there is also the major market to consider of veterinary services you provide.

A marketing plan is needed to try and obtain this share of the market (and then to keep it) and each practice will devise the plan and strategies to suit their circumstances. Points to consider include:

- client education
- client information
- producing a leaflet
- handing the leaflet to each client that comes through the door
- the receptionist asking each owner 'When did you last worm your pet?'
- the vets asking each owner 'When did you last worm your pet?'
- target mailings
- general mailings
- press advertising
- waiting room posters
- special offers or promotional offers.

The cost of promotions or special offers has to be borne by the increased turnover and profits generated as a result of the promotion. The process must then be reviewed and monitored to see if it was effective or ineffective, and the review will decide what lessons could be gleaned for future use. Similar market assessments can be made for veterinary services such as booster vaccinations, animals to be neutered, and annual health checks.

Your external and internal audit may illustrate a gap in the market for a 'specialist' in the practice and you may decide to offer a second opinion service to neighbouring practices.

Cost centre analysis

Cost centre analysis can be used to establish if you want to enter a particular market and also to help set proper fees that provide a realistic return on investment for the costs of the services provided.

If you wish to offer a cardiology service equipment will be needed such as scanners and printers, an ECG machine as well as good quality X-ray machines and laboratory facilities. Some of these may already be in the practice but need to be upgraded to reach a satisfactory standard for the work proposed. This frequently means new equipment has to be purchased and the capital costs should be included in the fee charged for provision of the service.

The inputs to this second opinion service must include training of the veterinary and non-veterinary staff involved as well as the set up costs. There may be equipment and possibly modifications to the premises plus an allocation of veterinary and nursing time and the associated administration time for reports and booking appointments.

Cost centre analysis allows you to cost all of the inputs accurately, including the set up costs, and ongoing cost and can be used to set correct fees for the services in question.

A similar assessment can be made for the veterinary services provided and the audit will indicate what percentage of your clients use your various services e.g. neutering, vaccination, dental care, clinics for adolescent, geriatric or obese pets.

The methods used and marketing plan to promote these services may be slightly different but reminders and recalls are easily produced from computer records held by the practice.

On the livestock side of the practice your audit should assess items such as:

- the number of livestock units
- the number of cows in the practice care
- the number of heifers in the practice care
- are they reared at home or away
- how many beef herds and calf rearers
- how many flocks of sheep and numbers
- calves and beef herds
- what are the confirmed diseases on each farm
- what is the current milk cell count on each unit
- what vaccination programmes are in place.

Farm reminders can be used for vaccinations but also for other areas such as worming reminders at turnout, housing and mid season, reminders for bolus wormers, lungworm vaccine and others.

There are many areas where good marketing will increase practice turnover and profit. The marketing plan is very important if you wish to achieve your aims. Marketing is fun, fulfilling and profitable.

Chapter 19
Record Keeping
Dixon Gunn

Keeping records is essential in financial terms but not all records are financially based.

Bookkeeping records may lay claim to being most important but before examining these consider the other records the practice should make and keep in order to run an efficient business:

❐ medical records
❐ policy records
❐ employment records
❐ business records
❐ bookkeeping records.

Medical records

These provide the history and outcome of cases. In small animal work it is worthwhile having individual records for each case, with each animal clearly identified. These should include:

❐ name
❐ breed
❐ age
❐ sex
❐ character: *Bites   Beware.*

In addition there should be notes on vaccination status, whether neutered or not, and a history of illness and treatment. If all these details are recorded then any veterinary surgeon can pick up the record, look at it and understand the animal about to be seen. Clients hate the attending veterinary surgeon not knowing about their animal.

In farm work, individual animals will not be recorded unless it is the history of, say, individual breeding cows or a special bull.

It is worthwhile keeping a farm record for each client. Just a date and a note of what was done, for example 'vaccinate herd against leptospirosis' or '1 May 2001: looked at 12 lame cows and advised on setting up a foot care system', and so on.

It is all too easy to forget what you said at the time unless you record it and you will need to be able to refer to these notes if the client sues the practice. If the client states that 'you never told me about looking after the cows' feet and look what happened' you need to be sure that the practice records can show that 'On 1 May 2001 I saw 12 lame cows and then set out for you a programme of foot care.'

Medical records are to help veterinary surgeons take over cases, to protect against untrue claims and also, if you are interested in carrying out research, they provide a database from which to start.

These medical records can be kept on computer or on cards. There are cards specifically designed for small animals or horses.

If you opt to keep your records on computer, then everyone in the practice has to know how to create new records and update existing records, and how to access them at any time. Medical records must be available to everyone involved at all times.

Policy records

The good practice will know how it wants to advise clients. It will have a policy on what to say to dog owners about vaccination and to farmers about preventive medicine. Each member of the practice must know the policy, so these decisions must be written down and be freely available to all staff. It is important that every member of staff who may be questioned by a client has the practice opinion available from which to quote.

Under policy records it is correct to include much more than just policy statements. Practice protocols, standard operating procedures and practice rules are all much the same type of document. In the contexts of COSHH and Care of Radiation, these documents are of great significance.

Employment records

A practice must keep records of disciplinary procedures, both verbal and written, and staff accidents. It must also provide every member of staff with a contract of employment setting out the terms of their employment, hours, wages, holidays, etc.

Business records

These are important documents. They are proof that you either own or have the lease of the premises. They prove an agreement with the bank to loan so much for so many years. They are proof of hire purchase agreements and lease purchase agreements.

Planning permission records are significant in purchase and sale of a practice and should be preserved with care.

Bookkeeping records

All practice financial activities must be recorded. At one extreme this is giving a secretary £5 to buy some coffee and on the other hand it might be recording that a client paid £5 for worm tablets for his dog. Equally it might be that £20 000 was paid for drugs supplied to the practice or that a client paid £1000 for services and drugs supplied in a given month.

Money received

The start is to keep records of money coming in to the practice. This comes from

❑ fees for services
❑ drugs sold.

The practice should be able to separate these two parts. It should know how much comes from each section. Further, if it is a mixed practice it should know how much comes from small animal fees and large animal fees, small animal drugs sold and large animal drugs sold. The ideal is to set up a system which allows the practice to record income under as many headings as it thinks necessary.

Keep records of all the money the practice receives, under as many sections as required. 'All money' includes consultancies and rents, as well as any other receipts. These records should also include the money the practice hopes to receive from accounts rendered.

A system of recording all income in a mixed practice might be as follows:

Large animal fees	
Small animal fees	
Government work	_____
Total fees	A
Large animal drugs	
Small animal drugs	_____
Total drug sales	B
Other receipts	C
	_____
Total practice income	(A + B + C)

This can be entered on a daily basis and from there it is totalled to provide a monthly figure. This figure includes both cash paid at time and money owed or on account. It is very important to divide the total into those two categories because bills have to be sent out promptly at the end of the month.

There is a pitfall to avoid. The total practice income should represent all the work done and drugs sold within a specific month. Do not include money received in the current month for work carried out and billed in the previous month. It is necessary to record that money has been received and the bill has been paid but this should be recorded separately from 'work done'. This is a debtors' record and it runs on month by month. This should be updated by adding on all the new accounts that have not been paid by the end of the month, and taking off all the old accounts that have been paid. The result is a new figure showing how much money the clients owe the practice at the end of the month.

Two separate records are required.

❐ *Practice turnover* is one record. This covers all the work done and drugs sold.
❐ *Book debt* is the second record. This shows how much has been paid to date and how much is still outstanding.

Expenditure

Every single penny should be recorded under the appropriate title: salaries and wages, drugs, telephone bills, insurance, etc. Again, record each invoice, whether or not it has been paid. In this way the record shows what has got to be paid out in the future.

The list of headings can be just as long as the practice wishes. For example if there are three cars, fuel costs of each car can be recorded, but avoid unnecessary detail. Partners' drawings and other expenses paid by the practice on behalf of partners must also be recorded.

There is also another category to consider: *capital expenditure*. Items such as an X-ray set or a new car are items of capital expenditure but they must still be included in the long list of expenditures – all part of record keeping.

Some costs can be grouped together for convenience, such as establishment costs and overhead costs. At the end of the month a list of costs can be drawn up under these headings.

Drug purchase
Salaries and wages
Establishment
Overheads
Motoring
Financial

Total costs   _____

Personal drawings
Capital expenditure

The timing of accounts to pay determines where they are placed in the record. Using the drug bill as an example, it will more than likely arrive about 4 April for all the drugs purchased in March. That bill goes into the March group because it is a debt incurred in March. It is not added in again in April when it is paid.

Financial costs must be carefully distinguished. For example interest paid on a loan is a financial cost; the capital of that loan is not – it is a *capital payment.* If in one month the practice pays interest of £100 and at the same time pays £1000 off the sum borrowed, the £100 is a financial cost and the £1000 is a capital payment and has to go into capital expenditure.

Above the line in the table everything is a month by month cost of the business and below the line it is in a different category. It may be thought that a partner's personal drawings are a cost of the business. They are not. They are available to the partner out of profits and they are only available if the profits are there.

If a system of recording all income and expenditure is set up, then after one short month the practice is well on its way to setting up management accounts which are of great value to both partners and the practice manager. (See Chapter 27 Management Accounts.)

Value added tax (VAT)

There is a statutory requirement to maintain records of all income and expenditure for VAT. The cash receipts and cheque payments records can provide this information but a separate VAT book should be kept to record details of monthly inputs and outputs, the VAT due for each quarter and the date of payment.

Summary

Record keeping in practice is a time-consuming duty. Some records can be updated and filed, for example planning permission details. Others, such as the financial records, must be continually updated. The secret is to update on a daily basis and to make use of the records to monitor practice performance.

Chapter 20
Stock Control

Dixon Gunn

'Stock in hand' is a phrase often used to describe the value of the drugs the practice has in stock at any one time. It is an odd phrase. In practice terms stock is not just any item which is purchased for onward sale to a client. There are many items which are used in the treatment of animals which are not specifically sold on. These are collectively known as *disposables*.

Examples of the first group, those for onward sale, are drugs, bandages, foods, orthopaedic implants and in today's small animal world, pet toys. The disposables are usually items such as disinfectants, cleaning materials, swabs and disposable syringes. But what of anaesthetics, X-ray developers, suture material, scalpel blades and so on? A useful definition of stock is 'all items which can be used only once by the practice in the provision of its services'.

Financial significance

It is important that a practice should realise the scope of its necessary purchases and equally recognise that quite a proportion of those purchases have to be absorbed within the fee charged for the service.

The percentage of gross turnover spent in purchasing 'stock' varies from about 27% in a small animal practice to about 38% in a practice only dealing with farm work. Because the majority of these purchases are sold on at a profit, the benefits to the practice, if handled correctly, are significant. Figures suggest that profit on drug sales is around 12% of turnover per veterinary surgeon in small animal practice and some 23% in large animal work. It is obvious from these figures that it is very important to handle stock correctly. After all, the drug bill is the single biggest account the practice has to face on a regular monthly basis.

Ordering stock

Because the account should be paid on time to benefit from discounts and the practice is aware of the date on which the account falls due, there is no need to run stock at a level which leaves the practice at risk of being unable to supply an item. This is not to say that purchases should fill up the shelves and wait for sales. The correct approach is to be able to forecast likely sales and maintain stocks to match levels of sales. Forecasting involves a practice history, modified by current activity and, as ever, a crystal ball.

Ordering requirements on a weekly basis improves use of staff time and makes it easier to set up a correct checking system. There will always be emergencies which can never be predicted and both wholesaler and manufacturers will respond immediately. The practice has to set levels of stock required to be held, based on a weekly ordering pattern. This must take into account the speed of turnover of the particular item. Twenty-five doses of canine vaccine in a predominantly small animal practice will probably be insufficient, whereas a single bottle of bovine leptospiral vaccine in the same practice could represent overstocking.

One reason for practices feeling that they must order 'on demand' (perhaps as often as five times a week) is justified by the practice saying that they do not have space to store more than one or two days of pet food sales. This puts the practice and the wholesaler under threat of failure to supply. If the business has grown in this way, then the practice should make appropriate arrangements for storage. If a system operates on a hand-to-mouth approach this always allows the possibility of slipping between the two.

Receipt of goods

In the ideal situation the practice drug and disposables order should be transmitted electronically to the wholesaler once a week. Upon receipt of the supplies, the following action trail should be carried out by the designated member(s) of staff.

(1) Check that goods supplied match invoice supplied.
(2) Check that goods supplied match goods ordered.
(3) Pass goods to practice pharmacy for storage.
(4) Note purchase price variations on previous price of each item.
(5) Implement increase in sale price immediately if there is any increase in purchase price. (This should include the sale price of items in stock.)
(6) Annotate invoice as verified and pass to accounts department for subsequent payment.

This is the method and even if it only involves one person, the routine should be the same every time. This is a perfect example of an SOP as discussed under policy records in Chapter 19.

Storage of goods (3) should be considered carefully. Obviously new supplies should be stored behind older supplies so that drugs are used in date order. Checking expiry dates of new supplies at this point is beneficial so that short dated stock can be identified and queried with the wholesaler if necessary.

Health and safety rules and Control of Substances Hazardous to Health (COSHH) Regulations must also be followed. Drugs and disposables can be toxic, inflammable, caustic, be classified as dangerous and, of course, are in fluid, powder, tablet and ointment form. Certain categories should be kept separate, for example inflammables, and fluids should not be stored above powders because of the risk of leakage.

Drugs may require to be kept at between 2°C and 8°C, in a dedicated refrigerator which is monitored to ensure that these limits are kept to.

Careful planning for the correct storage of all drugs is essential and access to the practice pharmacy should be restricted to those with a right and a need to enter.

Stocking levels

The number of items of each product which should be stocked varies with the frequency of use. All too commonly frequency of use, and therefore forecast of required stocking levels, are exaggerated. This leads to over-stocking and tying money up on the shelves. On average practices seem to carry about 50 days' worth of stock, worked out on the formula of:

$$\frac{\text{Value of stock in hand} \times 365}{\text{Annual stock purchase}}$$

Within this 50 day figure there will be stock which lasts ten days and some which lasts a year. It is worth investigating 'turn round' time of different types of stock as this improves the value of the forecast and the stock level.

With care, the stocking level should be reducible to 30 days. Some stock is purchased on the first of the month and paid for 45 or 50 days later; some stock is purchased on the last day of the month and is paid for 15 to 20 days later. On average stock is paid for 30 to 35 days after purchase, so a 30 day stock holding can mean that stock is sold before it is paid for.

Discounts and forward buying

The only worthwhile discount is a cash discount – more stock simply fills up the shelves. Cash discounts should be recognised as a reduction in purchase price, not an increase in turnover which is how they are wrongly recorded in some practice accounts.

It is only worth taking up the discount offer when the saving in purchase price is greater than the cost of tying up the money in the stock until it is sold. For example 5% discount on a £100 order equates with the cost of £95 tied up for 6.3 months at an interest rate of 10%. If the items cannot be sold and paid for in less than this time, the discount is not worth accepting.

Forward buying can come into a different category in that the practice accepts the stock but does not have to pay for it for a given period of time. As long as the amount of stock purchased is accurately forecast or there is a return agreement with the manufacturer, this method is beneficial.

Stock losses

Losses arise from breakages, contamination, allowing stock to go out of date and forgetting to record sales. It is this last item, forgetting to record sales, that costs practices large amounts of money every year. Only those practices with detailed stock control which can record the number of items bought against the number sold and correlate this with the number in stock can accurately determine their losses and take steps to minimise them.

Systems of recording at the time have to be set up and adhered to. The system can be paper invoice or electronic, including hand held terminals in cars, but the recording must be done at the time.

If an item costing £10 and selling at £15 is forgotten, the practice loses £5 of profit and £10 of costs. It has to sell two more items at £15 each to make the £10 of profit to pay for the cost of the forgotten item. The practice has bought three items, forgotten to record one and has to sell the other two to break even.

If the mark up is 20% rather than 50% as in the above example, the practice has to sell a further five items just to recover the cost of the forgotten item. There is still no profit.

Stock control in practice is essential for both the safe keeping of drugs and the financial success of the practice.

The method to use

Although a computer is not essential for effective stock control, it is certainly very useful, bearing in mind the detail involved.

The essentials for stock control are quite simple, they are only two in number:

- accurate recording of all product purchased
- accurate recording of all product sold or used in the provision of the service.

The difference between stock purchased and sold will provide the figure for stock in hand at any one time. Note that accurate recording poses great difficulties because in some situations, too many people are involved.

The first stage, that of reception of product should be restricted to a very small number of staff working under a very clear SOP.

The second stage, that of onward sale, is more difficult to control and the human error problem of forgetting to book sales by accident or even by design can never be discounted. As with reception of goods, a very few members of staff should be authorised to pass products from the pharmacy to other members of the practice and this includes partners.

The use of bar code readers by everyone in the practice is still a long way ahead but it might be the eventual solution. Computer records can only help when all personnel comply with practice protocols and feed in all necessary detail.

An audit over the year of items purchased and items sold or used will dramatically demonstrate the losses incurred by poor recording. The size of the loss suffered should be used as a spur to improve the quality of the practice records.

Chapter 21

Computers in Practice

Peter Gripper

The use of computers within practice and information technology (IT) is now so widespread all practices should address this subject and have an IT policy. It is not possible in a single chapter to cover all aspects of computers and I have restricted the text to their use, rather than their mechanics or to a list of equipment.

There can be few, if any, practices that no longer boast a computer or two on the premises. The real advantage of computers is what they can do for you and what benefits they offer.

For those who have an innate fear of computers, and often even for those who have an interest or love for computers, the best solution when considering IT and computerising the practice is to seek professional advice. The companies supplying advice will also usually supply equipment and it is essential that you establish a proper service and maintenance agreement. This agreement is of paramount importance in case the system fails for some reason or needs repair. The response time from engineers, provision of replacement equipment, repair times, modem 'fixes', and availability of telephone help lines all need to be considered. Be very wary of firms who only offer telephone helplines between 10.00 am–4.00 pm or only on premium rate telephone numbers.

There are some firms officially trained by the major software houses such as Microsoft, Sage and Lotus. A certificate of competence is only awarded to firms after they have been officially trained in the use of the software packages and systems. They are trained to put together compatible hardware and software packages for businesses after assessing your needs with you. The cost of systems sold by such companies is likely to reflect their input and service level.

As in many businesses the quality of equipment and service relates to price. Machines advertised in the high street, by mail order and by large discount retail outlets will often offer cheaper equipment but rarely any direct support. Shortcuts are available for the enthusiast and those 'in the know' who are prepared to undertake their own programme and software control but in the event of the system failing whilst that member of the practice is on holiday for two weeks then problems can arise.

There is a vast range of business software on offer from major software houses and in many respects the veterinary business is no different from any other business with regard to invoicing, banking, bookkeeping, or stock control. Off the shelf shrinkwrapped software that has already been tried and tested, and is regularly updated, has some advantages to offer over a specialist veterinary package, and the parent company may be more likely to be still around in ten years.

Clinical record systems for large or small animals are not readily available in the general market place and for this you will often need to look at a system adapted or designed for veterinary use. The bespoke veterinary systems often add a business package but the business element of the package may not be as user friendly or as versatile as the major software house's proven products.

Choosing a system

Before you look at systems it is advisable to write down full details of what you actually require – that is, what tasks do you want the system to undertake? This specification can be used when interviewing the companies to check that the services you want are actually available, and offered on the system that they propose to instal. It is worth recording these meetings and providing copies to the company so that there are no misunderstandings at a later date. With every system there will be some areas that are not as good as others and a balance has to be drawn between the versatility and the specificity of the system you opt for.

Unfortunately there is no guarantee that the company who sold you your system will remain in the same ownership or even in business, and you should look closely at the company before purchasing a system.

The type of computer system that suits your particular practice will vary but there are basic questions that will help you determine your requirements, such as:

❐ will it be used in consulting rooms?
❐ will it be used solely in the accounts department?
❐ how many consulting rooms are there?
❐ how many branch surgeries will it link to?
❐ how many office staff need a screen in front of them?
❐ how many workstations will be used at once?

In a small practice one or two PCs may meet the requirement and in a larger or multi-centre practice a network system with a central server and several workstations may be more appropriate. Some systems use modem links and others use a landline to ensure updated and current information is available at all sites. The speed of data transfer is important. The installation and maintenance costs of fixed landlines and ISDN lines is a major consideration that must be taken into account. Their operation to the standard you require should form part of the contract your supplier offers to you.

When choosing a system it is prudent to obtain some references from other practices who use the system and I suggest that part of the payment should be retained until the system is up and running. Always try and compare with someone who is using the system in the same way that you propose to use it. When you have a demonstration of the system, again ensure that the system that you see demonstrated is the same as the system that you are choosing. The old manual system (or the old computer) should always be run in tandem with the new system to ensure that it is working satisfactorily.

Maintenance for hardware and software is essential and it is important to find out what maintenance agreements are being offered. Not only is turn-out time important but also the repair time and provision of replacement machines whilst repairs are undertaken. Usually, if you pay an annual software support payment, you will receive free telephone advice and help, and also free correction of any 'bugs', frequently via modem. You should also get regular updates, either free or at cheaper rates.

In the event of a severe fire, flood or theft, your data is likely to be destroyed or lost and it is essential that proper back up procedures are followed. Information can be copied onto CD Rom, tapes or discs which should be stored away from the surgery. Back ups should be carried out automatically every day and some systems automatically back up information every fifteen minutes. This fear of losing everything dissuades many people from computerisation but the presence of a back up means the data can be restored which is more than can be said for most practice's paper record cards and account books in the event of a fire.

Computer viruses are hidden programmes that control some of your computer functions without your knowledge; they can slow the system down, stop it and in extreme cases erase data on the system. Anti-virus software should be installed at the outset and ensure a correct and proper procedure is established in the practice for virus checking. This is an increasing problem with machines now used by several people for different purposes and with different programmes. There is also the risk of collecting viruses from the internet or via e-mail.

Use of computers is no different to any other new technique and training is essential when installing a new system. Best results are obtained when proper training is provided for everyone on how to use the equipment. At some future stage further training will be advantageous to understand the refinements and more complicated tasks within the system. This is time consuming but essential and training is not cheap so check how much is included with your system purchase.

Use of computers

Computers have many uses that are varied and diverse and I have tried to illustrate some of them below. This is not intended to be an exhaustive list and the items are not in any particular priority order.

(1) Word processing and document production
(2) Stock management
    ❐ ordering

      ❐ stock control
      ❐ dispensing and labelling
(3) Client records and clinical case records, including invoicing
(4) Practice management, marketing and analysis
      ❐ financial
      ❐ internal analysis
      ❐ marketing services and newsletters
(5) Other systems, e.g.
      ❐ fertility programmes such as DAISY
      ❐ dairy nutrition programmes
(6) E-mail and intranet
(7) Website advertising and internet access
(8) Commercial equipment where computer technology is used without you necessarily realising it or requesting it, such as electronic till or dry chemistry analysers and hand-held stocktaking equipment and scanners
(9) Spreadsheets
(10) Databases
(11) Desktop publishing
(12) CPD.

For letter writing and production of documents the computer as a word processor has all but replaced the typewriter. Internal documents and letters can be produced to a very professional standard and the availability of colour printers, desktop publishing packages and ready made artwork allow anyone to produce documents and presentations to a very high standard. This can include client mailings, circulars, newsletters, client advice forms or leaflets, promotional material, mail merging and production of standard internal practice forms.

Stock control has huge financial implications and is discussed in its own right elsewhere in this book. Ensuring you have adequate stocks to treat the cases you see is essential, but keeping three or four times your requirement is unnecessary and costly. The larger wholesalers and several private firms offer computerised systems for stock ordering, stock management and stock auditing. There are several different approaches to the same problem and new and further options and developments are likely in the foreseeable future to include additional information and to help record keeping and labelling.

Hand-held equipment that can be linked to the main surgery machines but can also be taken onto clients' premises offers great potential. Auditing and batch number recording systems are also available.

With regard to dispensing, the use of pre-printed labels produced directly from information entered in the consulting room has much to offer. The clarity of the typed labels, and ensuring correct information is on the label for the client to read is a definite advantage. If any particular instruction or warning regarding the product should be on the label these can be printed automatically which also helps comply with COSHH and health and safety regulations. Some systems allow the product category to be linked to each drug so that if a client requests a prescription only medicine (POM) product the computer will flag the item and indicate to anyone trying to prescribe it that it is POM, and so can only be dispensed with veterinary surgeon approval.

Meeting current medicines legislation requirements for recording data, dispensing records, practice audits, batch number recording, traceability and recalls, are areas where computer technology offers solutions.

Clinical records and client records are offered with bespoke veterinary packages and these usually include facilities to generate booster reminders, labelling programmes and other patient recall options. Information is entered in the consulting room or from a monitor keyboard elsewhere and is priced automatically. In the dispensary a label is produced for any medication prescribed and this can then be dispensed for the client to collect and pay for at the reception desk.

Appointments and appointment lists are produced with a record of the arrival time of each client. The screen in the consulting room allows the consulting veterinary surgeon to know who is waiting, for how long they have been waiting and the animal and owner's records are available for viewing.

With any such system there are a series of entry levels and passwords to restrict access. Whenever anyone starts to use the system they enter their password and are allowed access up to their level; junior members of the practice would have a lower security code and lower access level. This also prevents inadvertent adjustments to the main system by inexperienced staff. Financial data should be restricted to the practice manager and partners.

There are few practices that cannot justify computerisation and soon recoup their financial outlay in time and efficiency savings. By properly pricing small animal work using a computer or an electronic 'smart till' (rather than by the veterinary surgeon pricing by hand) practice turnover can increase immediately by up to 15% in some practices.

Several of the specialist veterinary packages offer the opportunity to review and analyse treatments and diagnosis. This analysis can be useful for clinical reviews and also for marketing services to a particular patient group. Analysis of the type of work done and the percentage of work income derived from each part of the practice, such as vaccinations or neutering is very useful. Similarly, analysis of each individual veterinary surgeon's work is also very useful, and often enlightening.

It is in the area of practice management that computers come into their own. They provide so much information at the press of a button that allows you to monitor the work closely and accurately and the business within the practice. This applies not just to financial functions but also to many other areas.

The obvious financial areas that benefit from computer control are:

- ❏ invoicing
- ❏ sales ledger
- ❏ purchase ledger
- ❏ nominal ledger
- ❏ VAT returns
- ❏ monthly management accounts
- ❏ budget forecasts
- ❏ cash flow forecasts
- ❏ bank reconciliations
- ❏ payroll programmes for larger practices
- ❏ direct payments BACS/Autopay
- ❏ direct on-line banking.

Invoicing work is of paramount importance and providing the client with an invoice gives the impetus to pay. The ideal situation is where records are entered in the consulting room and labels are then automatically generated in the dispensary, and an invoice produced at reception which is presented to the client for payment. For farm clients, monthly accounts are more common and work is regularly entered during the month with invoices produced and mailed on the first or second day after month end. Prompt invoicing results in prompt payment.

The practice manager will find the information available on the system most useful when analysing practice records. For example monitoring the turnover per branch, per vet, per day, and examining many financial ratios such as sales of drugs compared to services, and income and expenditure analysis, as well as average transaction fees. This is particularly useful in analysing and understanding how practice income is generated and how to control expenditure.

Analysis of turnover per vet per month is always interesting in a practice and it is useful to know who is generating the income, particularly if salaries or bonuses relate to turnover. This information may be a rude awakening for some individuals but the positive side is that often the person who is the high income generator has a different approach, from which other vets can learn.

Once all the daily financial data is installed, the machine should produce monthly management accounts and VAT returns in a matter of moments. The end of year figures can be generated for your accountant which will save them duplicating the work, thus saving you money.

With monthly or quarterly management accounts you will also have good budget control and a realistic cash flow forecast to look at. This information is an essential management tool when considering the success of the business and allows a great deal of flexibility when planning and determining your borrowing requirements.

Many internal analyses are possible with computers that would be too laborious to calculate by hand. The availability of good accurate factual information allows you to make decisions that can result in real improvements. It is in this area that spreadsheets and databases are invaluable as a method of analysing vast amounts of data. Many calculations can be linked through the spreadsheet, using formulas, thus providing a very powerful analysis tool which will provide answers in seconds that would have taken several hours to calculate by hand. Modern software allows the operator to apply 'what if' scenarios to the figures on a spreadsheet. This can then be used to predict what would happen if, for example, turnover increased by 10% or if fees were increased by 3%, or both.

The effects on budgets and cash flow can be illustrated easily and the information used in decision making and planning. The 'what if' scenario can also be used the other way round to help determine at what level to set the practice fees to generate a particular net profit. Several different scenarios can be easily compared.

Not all calculations are financial, some are logistical. A simple analysis of the number of consultations per day showed us that 50% of the weekday consultations were carried out on Monday and Friday with the other 50% spread over the Tuesday, Wednesday and Thursday. This has obvious implications for staffing levels, when planning consultation hours within premises, and deciding whether to offer different consulting hours on different days. The large supermarkets analyse turnover per hour. Better planning gives better results.

From the marketing point of view the information is useful to help understand your customers and create a database of your customers and business. On the cattle and equine side of the practice it is useful to know how many animals are at each farm or stables and when routine procedures, e.g. boosters are due. The database can build up into full details of the routine drugs used or permitted on that unit, e.g. for drying off cows, which vaccines are used, how many youngstock there are and which services that client uses from the practice. Once you have the information to hand – and most of it is already in your files – you can use it to market your services or produce reminder letters.

Mailmerging and client address label printing means the work involved is minimal and not only are reminders sent on time but also you can offer some of your other services to those of your clients who do not already use them.

On the small animal side booster reminders are routine but also 'recalls' of other items are possible. The selection could be made by species, or by age or geographical region or by gender, or several of these combined and then be linked to mailmerged form letters so that a group of clients can be written to and invited, for example, to a local meeting in their area that relates to their pets. This form of target marketing uses your resources better and is far more likely to gain returns.

In equine practice the information collated would link owners with their animals and also with the stables at which they are kept. Then if the animal changes owner or the owner changes stables the information remains current. Frequently horses are sold within the geographical area and in this case, with the vendor's permission, the previous records could be transferred. When you plan to visit a particular yard you can check which horses are there and whether any of them are in need of routine treatment for example vaccinations, whilst you are there.

Computer law

Computer software is licensed for each user and if you pass on the programme to others you are breaking the law. The licence agreement is determined by the software manufacturer and will vary with how many machines you wish to install and the system you use.

The Data Protection Act is intended to protect any individual who is living and identifiable from unauthorised disclosure or abuse of data that has been recorded. Anyone storing records and personal information on computer about clients and their animals will need to register or else they are committing an offence and can be prosecuted. The Office of the Data Protection Register can be contacted at PO Box 66, Wilmslow, Cheshire SK9 5AX.

Future developments

The computer future holds great promise for businesses and also for veterinary science and education. Predicting progress is not easy but several ideas are now possible and I include a few thoughts below on what may be commercially available soon.

The improvement in portable laptop computers and printers means that it is now possible to carry a palmtop or laptop machine in the car with the practice system installed and a portable printer. When 'on-farm' it is simple to produce invoices the moment the work is finished using automatic pricing for any medicines used. The information can be backed up onto the main surgery machine. If this reduces the amount of unbooked drugs then it should pay for itself in the first year.

A lot of the exciting prospects relate to the great improvement in communication and the easier access to vast amounts of information from your own computer via a modem. Many practices and individuals at home use e-mail (electronic mail) and fax modems allowing transmission of documents via telephone lines. Transmission is very fast and information is received into your own computer and can then be called onto the screen or printed out.

The internet is growing with more users and international communication is now a reality for many computer users. There is access to vast amounts of information around the world and practices have their own websites for clients to browse through. These can be anything from a simple page with details of how to contact the practice through to photographs of each room and the staff and the chance to 'walk' into the practice and look round.

Internal websites, an *intranet*, purely for internal use within the practice is a good way of storing information and allowing easy access from workstations within the practice. This could be used for easy access to practice policy documents, health and safety data, price lists and an internal memo system or discussion board. In larger practices with more than one premises it offers an excellent communication and reference system.

Developments allow vast amounts of information to be stored on a single CD ROM, or on digital audio tapes (DAT), which can provide quick access to scientific references and global abstract searches from your own computer. The CD ROM offers interactive learning with pictures and videos to enhance any text and can be used as a reference source as part of the practice library.

Second opinion clinical systems, via websites, may be able to assist you with your diagnosis and offer examples of other cases. The 'diagnostic computer' is not going to replace clinicians but the access to current and accurate information will always be a boon to the progressive practice and an excellent reference source.

E-mail allows laboratory and other reports to arrive quickly into the practice and be in a format that can be easily added to the client records.

Optical character recognition (OCR) software, in conjunction with scanners allow documents to be scanned into your machine and be available as text documents that you can edit. All incoming mail could be scanned into your computer as you head towards the paper free office. Voice recognition programmes are available to turn your dictation into text on screen for you to send as a letter or report.

There are many more developments to come and they are not just for fanatics but have practical and often financial benefits to the practice.

Chapter 22
The Business Plan

John Gripper

When you start a new business and need to raise finance, your bank manager will ask to see your business plan. This will set out the aims and objectives of your business projected forward over the next few years.

A business plan is just as important for an existing business which should be planning for future events rather than just reacting to outside circumstances and drifting from one crisis to another.

The business may be a large veterinary manufacturing or wholesale company which would probably work to a five or ten year plan. It could be a veterinary school, a research establishment or an organisation like the Royal College of Veterinary Surgeons or the British Veterinary Association.

All veterinary practices – from the very large mixed practice to the one person small animal practice should have their own business plan.

The starting point of such a plan is to find out the answer to these fundamental questions.

- *Where are you now?*
- *Where would you like to be and when?*
- *How can you get there?*

Whilst this is a logical order to set out the questions, in many businesses the need for forward planning is only recognised when people wish to change so the question 'where would you like to be?' is often the first to be answered. This is an easy trap to fall into as a failure to first analyse your current situation can lead to internal discord and bad decision making.

Where is your practice now?

First you should carry out a detailed assessment of your present financial position as shown in the practice profit and loss accounts and the balance sheet. This will need to be supplemented by further financial information on the current value of practice assets, a division of income on a species and individual veterinary surgeon basis, and also on fees received for services as compared to the sale of drugs.

A further breakdown of income from services can then be made so that for a small animal practice an assessment could be made of its case load of consultations, operations, vaccinations and average transaction fee, etc.

Practice costs also need to be broken down into the following six broad categories:

- Drugs
- Motoring
- Overheads
- Salaries and wages
- Establishment
- Finance

Once this background of financial information has been obtained then the practice should compare itself to other similar practices in type of work and geographical location by use of the median figures from the annual BVA/SPVS survey. This will give an indication of relative profitability and efficiency of the different aspects of the practice and also the return on capital investment.

This financial analysis is the necessary starting point for future planning but it is only a base measuring device to allow future monitoring of the plan. Most planning involves conceptual thinking, not number crunching.

The next stage is a general assessment of the practice and here there are advantages in using an experienced management consultant to help with this assessment. An outsider can give an objective overview, introduce fresh ideas and avoid existing personality conflicts. With an outside consultant the staff often feel more free to talk openly about the problems and their perception of the business.

The consultant who helps form the business plan need not have a great depth of knowledge of veterinary practice although if a suitable consultant is available with experience of veterinary practice this would be an advantage. He or she should act as an independent chairman to guide the discussions and not try to impose their views on the practice.

This general assessment is carried out by a series of interviews with the partners and all senior staff members including the veterinary assistants, practice manager, nurses and reception staff. These interviews are conducted on a 'one to one' basis and also by small group discussions. A technique often used in the discussions at this stage is called SWOT analysis which determines the practice in relation to its:

- *Strengths*: the positive aspects of the practice
- *Weaknesses*: the skill gaps
- *Opportunities*: where improvements can take place
- *Threats*: the potential or actual business risks

Following this series of interviews and discussions, the consultant then prepares a paper which gives a summary of the existing position of the practice and tries to get general agreement on the answers to the question '*Where are we now?*'.

Where does the practice want to be and when?

The first task should be an examination of the philosophy of the practice and the restating of it. Mission statement, practice culture, call it what you like, it will be an overriding vision or purpose that will permeate through the plan with all key objectives reflecting it.

Your practice statement should be short and concise – a single sentence is often adequate, for example:

> 'To expand the practice, improve its profitability and enhance its reputation by increasing the range of skills and specialised expertise available to provide a high standard of animal care'.

Having established comparative ratios and financial criteria against which the planning can now be assessed, it is now possible to set out the strategic objectives.

In setting objectives some assumptions will need to be made and these should be as simple as 'no new practice setting up in the area' or that the 'rate of inflation remains in the range of 3% to 5%'. These simple assumptions should all be written down as the plan is a working document subject to periodic review and updating.

On the basis of the information already obtained on the current position there should now be a longer term look into the future and this can best be obtained by a brain storming session in which lots of ideas are thrown about and freely discussed by selected groups of personnel within the practice.

The main issues and problems will need to be identified and a number of discussion sessions may have to be held in order to reach general agreement on alternative options to determine the future objectives of the practice. These sessions will be led by an experienced consultant who may use visual aids and other techniques to help control the group and channel discussion into positive conclusions.

The focus of these discussions will be the SWOT analysis. The practice should build on its strengths and seek to remedy its weaknesses, opportunities should be explored and countermeasures prepared against the threats. Here are some examples of the areas that may need to be looked at.

- future capital investment into buildings and equipment
- siting and status of practice premises
- future size and staffing of practice
- partnership structure
- advertising and marketing of services
- purchase and sale of drugs
- stock control
- fee levels
- computerisation
- motor vehicles – type and size
- potential for growth in different areas and species
- setting up practice laboratory
- specialisation
- diversification into new areas of work

How do we get there?

Having set practical and clear cut objectives for the future, the next step of the business plan is to determine how things are to be achieved and who is to be responsible for their implementation.

Whilst general assumptions have been made when setting the future objectives another set of criteria begins to emerge at this stage. These are the *critical issues* or *critical success factors* – that is the major matters that will alter your ability to achieve your objectives.

Critical success factors differ from assumptions in so far as assumptions are realistic conclusions based on the best information available at the time, whilst critical issues *must* or *must not* happen for the planned objectives to be achieved and are not always predictable, for example, planning permission is refused for the proposed new branch surgery, or the current partnership is dissolved.

A core part of any business plan is the institution of a budget forecast which will set out the expected turnover, costs and profitability. This should be supported by monthly management accounts so that the financial position of the practice can be accurately monitored on a regular basis, by comparing the monthly figures to the budget forecast figures.

Additional staff training may be required in order to obtain greater expertise and skills to develop the plan.

Another acronym which is used at this stage of business planning is called the SMART analysis:

❏ Specific
❏ Measurable
❏ Actionable
❏ Realistic
❏ Timed

In other words the plan now has to be clearly defined into different areas and made into an action plan with specific tasks delegated to named individuals in the practice, who will each be required to make regular progress reports at future practice meetings.

The targets must be measurable and constantly reviewed. The time scale has to be laid down in a realistic manner so that the targets are achievable; however the agreed time scale or objectives may require adjustment. In all business plans there has to be a flexibility to allow for changes due to circumstances outside the control of the practice.

The final business plan should contain the following:

(1) *A vision for the future* – this is a sense of mission with a picture of what can be achieved.
(2) *Strategies and objectives* – this is the translation of the vision into specific long term statements of the objectives, strategic options, action programmes and budgets.

(3) *Establishment of values and ethics* – each practice has its own distinctive character, style and culture and these values are based on the personalities and successes of its members.
(4) *Policies and priorities* – a concise summary of the overall plan which can be circulated to all staff so that everyone in the practice can understand and follow future policies.
(5) *Obtaining resources* – this will cover both training and motivation of staff and also the obtaining of financial resources.
(6) *Monitoring achievement and performance* – regular monitoring of performance is necessary to ensure that forecasts and objectives are being met.
(7) *Approval of plans* – the business plan must be based on a consensus view and agreed and approved by all senior practice members.

Chapter 23

Understanding Practice Accounts

John Gripper

Choose your practice accountant with care. Often the choice will be between the small town firm, where you are more likely to receive personal attention from a known individual, or one of the large national accountancy partnerships.

It is preferable to employ an accountant who already has experience of veterinary practice accounts. A good accountant should not only prepare your annual accounts within a reasonable period of time from the end of your financial year, but should provide you with general financial and tax advice – at a reasonable fee.

The full auditing of accounts is expensive and only necessary if you are a limited company whose turnover exceeds £350,000, and you could, if you wished, prepare your own practice accounts. However, home produced practice accounts are more likely to be subject to close scrutiny by the Inland Revenue than a set of accounts produced by a known firm of accountants whom the Inspector of Taxes has come to respect and trust.

Your accountant will normally include a covering statement with the accounts such as:

> 'In accordance with the instructions given to us, we have prepared, without carrying out an audit, the annexed accounts for the year ending 31 December 2000 from the books and records of the veterinary practice and from information and explanations supplied to us and confirm that in our opinion the accounts are in accordance therewith.'

The wording of this statement does not imply that your accounts are not correct – it is simply terminology used by accountants to protect themselves against the discovery at a later date that you have not been completely honest over your disclosures.

In this chapter you will find a sample set of practice accounts for Messrs Dolittle and Dalley, veterinary surgeons who run a three person mixed practice composed of two partners and employing a veterinary assistant.

Messrs Dolittle and Dalley, MRCVSs
Veterinary Surgeons

Contents

Profit and loss account at the year ending 31 December 2000

Schedule of fixed assets as at 31 December 2000

Balance sheet as at 31 December 2000

Schedule of partners' capital accounts as at 31 December 2000

Statement of source and application of funds

Profit and loss account

	£	2000 £	£	1999 £
Income				
Fees		**310,000**		**288,000**
Cost of drugs	85,903		79,385	
Opening stock of drugs	7,000		6,000	
Closing stock of drugs	4,000	**88,903**	7,000	**78,385**
Gross profit		**221,097**		**209,615**
		(71.3%)		(72.7%)
Other receipts				
Bank deposit interest	100		200	
Rent	—	**100**	100	**300**
		221,197		**209,915**
Expenses				
Salaries				
Professional salaries	32,597		27,645	
Lay staff salaries	41,000	**73,597**	39,000	**66,645**
Motoring costs				
Garage charges	9,500		9,000	
Insurance and road tax	1,250		1,000	
Depreciation	4,750	**15,500**	5,000	**15,000**
Establishment costs				
Rents and rates	4,600		4,150	
Insurances	400		350	
Maintenance of premises	4,200		2,500	
Heating and lighting	3,800	**13,000**	2,500	**9,500**
Overheads				
Machine rentals	600		600	
Accountancy	2,000		900	
Legal	1,100		—	
Subscriptions	1,500		1,600	
Laundry and cleaning	500		500	
Postage	1,500		1,400	
Telephone	2,800		2,600	
Course fees	1,700		2,900	
Printing and stationery	1,400		1,800	
Sundry expenses	2,100	**15,200**	2,500	**14,800**
Financial				
Bank charges	1,900		1,600	
Interest paid	3,770		4,820	
Bad debts	2,200		600	
Depreciation	1,740	**9,610**	1,950	**8,970**
Net profit		**94,290**		**95,000**

2

Schedule of fixed assets as at 31 December 2000

Fixed assets	31/12/99	Additions	Disposals	Depreciation	31/12/00
	£	£	£	£	£
Property	80,000	50,000	—	—	130,000
Instruments and equipment	7,360	90	—	3,200	4,250
Fixtures and fittings	8,600	510		3,500	5,610
Motor vehicles	22,000	6,000	2,000	11,750	14,250
Goodwill	10,000	—	—	—	10,000
Wholesale company	880	—	—	—	880
Total	128,840	56,600	2,000	18,450	164,990

Depreciation	31/12/99	Depreciation	Adjustment on sale	31/12/00
Instruments and equipment	2,360	840	—	3,200
Fixtures and fittings	2,600	900	—	3,500
Motor vehicles	7,000	5,750	1,000	11,750
Total	11,960	7,490	1,000	18,450

Balance sheet as at 31 December 2000

	2000 £	1999 £
Fixed assets		
Property	130,000	80,000
Instruments and equipment	4,250	5,000
Fixtures and fittings	5,610	6,000
Motor vehicles	14,250	15,000
Goodwill	10,000	10,000
Shares in wholesale company	880	880
	164,990	116,880
Current assets		
Stock of drugs	4,000	7,000
Stock of stationery	200	400
Debtors	22,500	16,500
Payments in advance	700	600
Cash in hand	480	1,200
	27,880	25,700
Current liabilities		
Creditors	15,000	15,500
PAYE and VAT	4,200	3,800
Bank overdraft	—	1,500
Mortgage	4,000	4,000
Long term liabilities		
Business loan	23,000	30,000
	46,200	54,800
Net assets	146,670	87,780
Financed by capital accounts		
Balance at 1 January 2000	87,780	81,750
Net profit for the year	94,290	95,030
Revaluation of property	50,000	—
Less drawings	85,400	91,000
	146,670	85,780

4

Schedule of partners' capital accounts as at 31 December 2000

	D. Dolittle	I. Dalley	Total
	£	£	£
Balance at 1 January 2000	57,780	30,000	87,780
Net profit share	42,756	42,756	85,512
Interest on capital	5,778	3,000	8,778
Revaluation of property	25,000	25,000	50,000
Total	131,314	100,756	232,070
Less drawings	32,000	38,000	70,000
Less income tax	6,400	6,000	12,400
Less private pension	2,000	1,000	3,000
Total	40,400	45,000	85,400
Balance at 31 December 2000	90,914	55,756	146,670

Statement of source and application of funds

Year ending 31 December 2000

	£	£
Bank overdraft		**(100)**
Profit for the year before partners' drawings	94,290	
Add depreciation	6,490	**100,680**
Other sources of funding		
Other long term funding	—	
Proceeds of sale of fixed assets	2,000	**102,680**
Application of funds		
Purchase of fixed assets	6,600	
Loan repayments	7,000	
Partners drawings	85,400	**3,680**
Movement in working capital		
(increase)/decrease in stock	3,200	
(increase)/decrease in debtors	(6,100)	
increase/(decrease) in creditors	(100)	**680**
Closing bank in hand/(overdraft)	480	
Increase/(decrease) in working capital		**1,160**

6

Profit and loss account

All figures shown in the profit and loss account (also called the income and expenditure account) will be exclusive of value added tax. The practice income is shown at the top of the sheet and all the expenses are then listed and subtracted from the income to show a figure for net profit at the bottom of the page.

The item for gross income represents fees from veterinary services and the sale of veterinary medicines carried out by the practice. Many of the figures shown on the profit and loss account can be used for direct comparison with the previous year's, and also with other practice statistics.

The other item of income is *other receipts* which will be non-veterinary in origin such as rent, commission, dividends, interest on bank deposit or building society accounts. Manufacturers and wholesalers discounts received in respect of drug purchases should not be shown as income but deducted from the cost of drugs.

In these accounts the turnover showed a rise of 7.6% over the previous year as compared with a rise of 3% in RPI (Retail Price Index). The turnover per veterinary surgeon was £103 333 which was lower than the 1999 Survey figure for mixed practices of £128 750. The average cost of drug purchases per veterinary surgeon was £29 634 as compared with a Survey figure of £40 128 for mixed practices.

The gross profit (turnover less drugs) is 71.3% which is lower than the previous year. Care must be taken when comparing gross profit figure between practices as some accountants deduct salaries and wages and the cost of laboratory charges to arrive at a figure of gross profits.

Expenditure

It becomes clear that the figure for the closing stock of drugs will have a direct effect on profit i.e. if the closing stock was £3000 higher then both the gross and the net profit would increase by the same amount. For this reason a full stocktake of the drugs and disposables should be undertaken at the end of each financial year – and that should include any drug stocks in the cars. Most practices carrying out this stocktaking exercise for the first time will be surprised at how high their stock levels are. In mixed practice we expect stock levels to be between 30 and 40 days of annual purchase.

The other main categories of expenses are for convenience divided into five main groups: salaries and wages, motoring costs, establishment costs, overheads and financial costs.

The salaries and wages should be divided into those paid to professional staff, i.e. veterinary assistants and locums, and those paid to the lay staff. These figures should include employer's National Insurance contributions and also the cost to the practice of assistants' accommodation.

Motoring costs will include all the actual car running expenses, i.e. road tax, car insurance, petrol, tyres, repairs and also car depreciation. If the cars are leased then the leasing charges will also be entered into this section. If the cars are owned by the partners then the mileage payments paid to the partners should be included. You can calculate the actual cost per mile by dividing the motoring costs by the total car mileage and see how your figures compare to the current MAFF mileage rate.

The establishment costs are those costs that are necessary to maintain the surgery premises, i.e. rent, heat, light, rates, surgery insurance, maintenance and repair of the premises.

The overheads will include all the other practice expenditure apart from the financial items. The main costs will be equipment leasing, subscriptions, laundry and cleaning, postage, packing and carriage, telephone, course fees, printing and stationery, advertising and sundry expenses.

The financial costs will be bank charges i.e. commission and interest, mortgage and loan interest, bad debts, depreciation of equipment, instruments, and fixtures and fittings. The figure for bad debts will be the amount of debt written off during the year as irrecoverable and a provision may be made for possible bad debts that may be written off in the future.

All these costs should be compared with the previous year to see if they are rising faster than the increase in turnover on a percentage basis. Some costs such as rates will be fixed while others such as telephone, heating and lighting will be variable and related to throughput of work.

The bottom line is the figure for net profit. This is the figure that will be used as a basis for income tax but adjustments will have to be made for depreciation and capital allowances before arriving at the taxable profit for Schedule D.

The percentage of net profit to turnover can be calculated but when comparing your net profit with other practices remember to make sure that you are comparing like with like. For example:

Do you pay partners' wives a salary and pension premiums?
Do the partners run one or two cars each and are the running costs put through the practice?
Do the partners have high overseas congress expenses?

Schedule of fixed assets

The detailed valuation of the property, cars, veterinary instruments, equipment, fixtures and fittings and computers, and the depreciation of these assets that has been deducted during the financial year is shown on the schedule of fixed assets. Depreciation of 25% to $33\frac{1}{3}\%$ may be claimed on these assets but the capital allowance for income tax is set by the Inland Revenue.

Additions and deductions that have taken place during the year are taken into account before depreciation is deducted so as to arrive at the net book figure at the end of the financial year.

A balancing charge applies when a motor vehicle or piece of equipment is sold and the proceeds exceed the written down value. The 25% annual writing down allowance may not be appropriate for some equipment called 'short life assets' such as computers that need to be written off during their expected short working life. The capital allowances of these short life assets that are expected to be redundant within three to five years of acquisition will have to be calculated separately on a straight line basis over a short period.

Balance sheet

The capital employed in the practice is shown on the balance sheet which lists all the assets and the liabilities. One of the major assets will be the property. The property may show an appreciation or depreciation in value and it might be advisable that every two or three years a realistic value should be shown in the accounts for the practice property.

A revaluation of the property can be carried out by the partners themselves. However if there is a change of partnership in the practice, a professional valuation should be obtained from a qualified estate agent or chartered surveyor. A property revaluation in the accounts will not involve the practice in any extra tax liability, but it does strengthen, on paper, the total value of the assets and this could be useful when the practice is approaching a bank or other financial institution to arrange an overdraft or loan.

It is not always considered necessary to show goodwill as an asset; but if goodwill has recently changed hands then it is sometimes included as a fixed asset. The date should be shown when the last goodwill valuation was carried out.

The figure for debtors is the amount owed to the practice by the clients at the end of the financial year; compare this figure to the previous year to establish a trend and also calculate the average number of days that the debtors take to pay their accounts:

$$\frac{\text{Total debtors} \times 365}{\text{Turnover less cash takings}} = \text{Average number of days for collection of debts}$$

In this calculation it is important to subtract the cash takings from the turnover in order to arrive at an accurate figure for the debt collection time. If in your practice the number of days is higher than 40 for the collection of debts then your credit control needs tightening up.

It is important to emphasise again that the figure for drugs stocks should reflect the current value of the drugs on the shelves and in the cars and this should be carried out by a physical stocktake each year. A mixed practice will usually carry 5 to 6 weeks' supply of drugs and a small animal practice about 4 weeks' supply – so that a rough estimate of your stock levels can be obtained by dividing the annual purchase of drugs by 9 for a mixed practice and 12 for a small animal practice. To calculate the number of days for the turnover of stock, use the following formula:

$$\frac{\text{Stock levels} \times 365}{\text{Annual drug purchases}} = \text{Average number of days for stock turnover}$$

The figure for creditors represents the money that the practice owes to its suppliers. Most drug wholesalers offer discount for prompt payment by a specified date. It makes good sense to pay local suppliers on time to ensure that your garage, plumber, electrician, etc., provide you with a prompt service. Rates, gas, electricity and telephone bills can always be left until the red notice and the adventurous can stretch their PAYE, VAT and income tax payments to the maximum limits before incurring interest and penalties, although this is not to be recommended.

Payments in advance refer to items, such as insurance for property or professional indemnity, which are paid in advance on an annual basis.

Loans should always be shown as liabilities but some accountants may show long term loans with repayments over a period of a year as a separate entry.

Schedule of partners' capital accounts

Partners' capital accounts show the individual breakdown of the partners' holdings in the capital of the partnership. Sometimes the partners' holdings are shown in two accounts: the *capital* account and the *current* account, or these may be merged together.

The capital account represents the investment in the practice including any increase or decrease in the property revaluation. The current account is used to show the partners' net profit for the year added to the previous balance less the partners' drawings and their personal income tax, National Insurance and personal pension deductions.

A difference between these two accounts may arise where one partner has a larger shareholding of the practice property or if one partner has withdrawn a disproportionate share of the practice profits. If there are unequal capital holdings between the partners it is only fair that these should be adjusted to compensate the partner who has the greater share of the practice capital.

The calculation of *interest on capital* can correct any differences in the amounts of the capital accounts and the interest adjustments credited to the partner before the division of profits – however it is part of the profits and not counted as unearned income. The notional rate of interest is usually linked to the average bank base rate for the financial year. You can obtain this figure from your bank.

A notional interest rate of 10% was used in our sample accounts. Too high a notional rate of interest may encourage partners to leave excess capital in their capital account just to earn more than the market rate of interest.

Unequal capital holdings can also be a useful way of allowing a new partner to join a partnership – he or she can come in on an equal profit sharing basis but initially does not have to put in an equal amount of capital as the existing partners. Over the years he can gradually build up his capital account by drawing less than the other partners.

If full drawings are taken each year then the working capital will have to be funded from elsewhere. An expanding practice in an inflationary climate will need to retain capital each year to finance its higher drug stocks, increased debtors, new veterinary instruments and equipment, improvements to properties and purchase more expensive motor cars. This can be funded by the partners agreeing to leave a percentage of profits (say up to 10%) in the practice each year to provide finance for the extra working capital that is required.

Statement of source and application of funds

The statement of source and application of funds ('source and ap') is much loved by younger accountants. It shows the changes in your liquid assets during the year. A decrease is bad news as it means that the practice is underfunded. This can be corrected internally by a restriction on partners' drawings, or funded by the introduction of new capital.

An increase is good news as it means that a surplus of money has been generated during the year which would allow the partners to withdraw some of their capital or to invest in better equipment or improve their properties.

To determine the source of funds in our example, you start with any negative cash assets such as a bank overdraft, and then add the profit for the year and also the depreciation. The depreciation figure is added back because it is only an accounting book figure and it does not involve the actual movement of money. Other additions will be any extra funding or the sale of assets.

The 'application of funds' shows where the money has been spent and will be used for the purchase of fixed assets, loan repayments and partner drawings. There then has to be an adjustment for the movement of working capital in respect of drugs, debtors and creditors. An increase in stock and debtors is negative cash flow as they take money out of circulation. An increase in creditors is positive cash flow as it retains money within the practice.

Finally the closing cash in hand (or overdraft) is taken into consideration. The total for the source of funds is added together and the total for the application of funds is subtracted to determine if there has been an increase or decrease in working capital at the end of the year.

Whilst our example shows that there has been only a modest increase in working capital it should be pointed out that the practice had also been able to repay £7000 of a business loan during the year.

Summary

Practice accounts have to be prepared so that the net profit and the capital allowances for Schedule D income tax and Class 4 National Insurance contributions can be calculated and agreed with the Inspector of Taxes.

Under the new self assessment system that was introduced for the 1996/7 tax year there is a change from the preceding year basis to the current year basis of assessment.

Although by the time you receive your annual accounts many of the figures are well out of date they are a very useful source of information for comparison with your previous year's figures and also with other veterinary practices of a similar type by means of the BVA/SPVS annual survey.

If you wish to expand the practice and arrange further borrowings then your bank manager will wish to study your sets of practice accounts to establish your profit record over the years and assess your ability to maintain loan repayments in the future.

Internal management accounts will be needed to monitor your up-to-date performance as your year end accounts will only provide a historical record of your practice but the information in the annual accounts can be a very useful guide in the preparation of your future budget forecasts.

Chapter 24
Budget Forecasts and Performance Monitoring
John Gripper

The philosophy of budgeting is to turn your long term plans into actual figures which will set targets for future business performance. Monitoring the actual performance against the budget will allow early detection of problems and deficiencies.

Budgeting should involve all senior members of the business and 'bottom up' budgeting starts at managerial or departmental levels and works upwards to the owners or directors, setting profit levels. Once budgets have been agreed then these are an effective tool for the efficient running of the business through the delegation of authority within set budgets.

Budget preparation

(1) Set *guidelines* and *objectives* which will be in accord with the current business plan. For example, to open up a new branch surgery or start marketing petfoods.

(2) Make certain *assumptions*. This will be your best economic guesstimate as to what is likely to be happening in the country next year, i.e. rate of inflation, bank borrowing interest rate and average wage inflation.

(3) Forecast *sales* and *activity* levels in your practice which should reflect the real growth of the business in terms of throughput and volume of drug sales.

(4) Forecast gross *income* from your expected growth in sales and activity levels plus adjustments for fee and drug price increases.

(5) Estimate *costs*. Some of your costs will be variable and directly related to activity, for example the sale and use of drugs relates to throughput of cases. Other costs which do not have a direct relationship to your turnover, will be fixed such as rates or insurance premiums. Remember to include a contingency item for the unexpected costs.

(6) You should determine a realistic level of *profit* that the partners should aim to achieve in the forthcoming year.

A continuing business will be able to utilise current information from their management accounts to help forecast income and expenditure but a new business just starting up will have to begin with a blank piece of paper.

Cash flow forecast

Cash flow is much loved by bank managers as it predicts the size of the bank overdraft required over the year on a month to month basis. For a new practice it is an essential exercise but for the existing practice that has established good credit and overdraft facilities it is of less importance.

In order to construct your cash flow forecast you take the figures of income and expenditure which you have estimated for your annual budget and allocate them over the next twelve months.

Some payments such as insurance may be paid annually and others such as gas, electricity and telephone are paid quarterly. Value added tax should be included but not depreciation or bad debts where no movement of cash takes place.

Once you have divided the annual expenditure into each month you follow the same process for income but remember to allow for any seasonal variation, i.e. small animal work is busier in the summer, calving in the autumn, and lambing and equine stud work in the spring.

A start up practice will be asked to prepare an income forecast and cash flow for the first three years on the basis of an estimated number of consultations, operations and visits, with average fees for each procedure. If all goes well a new practice can expect a build up of work to the level of a one man practice within three years of start up.

Your cash flow will predict the level of available cash in the practice bank account which helps you determine the best time to undertake capital expenditure such as property improvements or the purchase of new cars and equipment (See Table 24.1). A more extensive discussion of cash flow is to be found in Chapter 26.

Table 24.1 Cash flow for each month.

	January	February	March	April	May
	(£)	(£)	(£)	(£)	(£)
Income	10,000	11,500	14,500	13,500	16,000
Expenditure	11,500	8,500	12,500	14,000	12,800
Net + or (–)	(1,500)	3,000	2,000	(500)	3,200
Bank balance	(1,500)	1,500	3,500	3,000	6,200

Budget timetable

Budget preparation should commence at least three months before the end of the current year. You can draw up the general guidelines, specific objectives and agree the assumptions. A detailed appraisal and draft budget can then be drawn up for approval by the partners. The assumptions, activity levels and level of net profit can be reviewed for the final budget which must be agreed by the end of the current year.

Monitoring performance

The final budget that has been agreed is for a full accounting year and must now be divided into a monthly basis so that it can be used for your monthly management accounting. This breakdown will involve making adjustments to the income for seasonal variation which will be known by past experience.

There will also be a known variation and pattern for costs which are not necessarily paid on an even monthly basis throughout the year. Some costs, like the purchase of drugs, will have a similar seasonal pattern as the throughput of work.

The monthly management accounts will show the actual financial performance and this should be compared to the budgeted figures, and on a monthly and a year to date (YTD) basis (see Table 24.2). Comparisons should also be made to the figures for the previous year.

Table 24.2 Cumulative year to date (YTD) comparison.

Month	Net profit (£)		% comparison	
	1998/9	1999/00	Month	YTD
April	4,278	5,543	129.57	129.57
May	5,768	5,878	101.91	113.69
June	3,387	4,238	125.13	116.57
July	4,996	4,667	93.41	110.29

The results can be displayed in graph form and many businesses use the moving annual total (MAT) as an ongoing indicator. The moving annual total is the last twelve months' performance. You start off with your previous year's annual total and add on the first month's figures and deduct the figures for the same month a year ago. This method eliminates seasonal fluctuations and the final figures can be tabulated or drawn in a graph from which by extrapolation you can predict your yearly figures (see Table 24.3).

Another method of assessing your performance is to express all your costs as a percentage of the turnover with the objective of trying to maintain or improve your practice cost ratios. Here the information from interpractice comparisons is invaluable. The BVA/SPVS Annual Survey allows you to compare your own practice figures as cost ratios as a percentage of total revenue with the median figure for similar types of veterinary practices (see Table 24.4).

Table 24.3 Moving annual total (MAT) comparison.

Month	Drug costs (£)		MAT
	1998/9	1999/00	£26,400
April	2,500	2,775	26,675
May	2,250	3,350	27,775
June	3,450	3,150	27,475
July	1,178	1,890	28,187

Table 24.4 Examples of cost ratios/total revenues from 1998 BVA/SPVS Survey for small animal practice in Midlands region.

Costs	% of total revenue
Drugs and disposables	26.83
Support staff	17.49
Motor	2.56
Establishment	3.78
Overheads	11.69
Professional	10.61
Net profit	26.06

Once the final annual budget has been agreed it should not be changed. All the differences between forecast and actual will be shown as variables and can be expressed in actual figures and percentage terms.

Summary

In order to run any business effectively you must be in financial control and this means that you must have accurate up to date information on the performance of the business. By waiting until your accountant has prepared your annual accounts you have delayed making decisions and taking corrective action in your business.

Decisions such as whether you can afford to employ another assistant, set up a branch surgery, the level of fee increases, whether to buy or lease cars or equipment, etc., are all dependent on having up to date financial information available.

Most budget forecasts can now easily be prepared by suitable accounting software packages and spreadsheets on your practice computer. This allows you to look at different options by asking the question 'What if?'.

However it is important that the preparation of the budget income forecasts and cash flows, followed by the monitoring through monthly management accounting, is carried out by the practice 'in house', rather than just handing over the responsibility to your accountant.

Chapter 25
Capital Budgeting
John Gripper

No business can afford to stand still. A veterinary practice, just like any other successful small business, must be prepared to progress by investing capital to expand and improve its facilities to provide benefits for the future.

An expanding business will also need to fund the increase in the value of the current assets shown on its balance sheet which may occur from an increase in the value of debtors and stock but which may be offset by higher creditors.

There are three main areas which require capital expenditure on fixed assets within a veterinary practice.

□ *Practice premises* – Existing premises may need to be improved or extended. Premises may be purchased to open a new branch surgery or a new veterinary small animal or equine hospital may be built.
□ *Equipment* – There will be a requirement to replace or upgrade X-ray machines, anaesthetic scavenging systems, laboratory test equipment, kennels and of course the practice motorcars. New modern diagnostic equipment such as endoscopes, electrocardiography and ultrasound machines may also need to be purchased.
□ *Cost reduction and improved efficiency* – This is where the purchase of new capital equipment could bring about a cost saving and improve the practice efficiency by the purchase of modern office equipment, a new computer system, intelligent till, fax machine, photocopier and mobile telephones.

Definition of capital expenditure

The purchase of an asset, such as a car or a building, is clearly capital expenditure. If a practice spends money with the intention of buying a capital asset, and does not succeed in the acquisition, that too will be classed as capital expenditure.

Money spent on improving a building or other asset will normally be regarded as capital expenditure and therefore disallowable for income tax purposes, whereas if money is spent on repairs, the expense will be tax allowable as a cost against practice income. Therefore the costs of decoration, repairs and maintenance of premises are fully tax allowable against any profits but any alterations, additions or improvements of business premises are regarded as non-deductible expenditure for tax purposes.

There may be a grey area when practice premises are modernised in the exact definition of *repairs* and *improvements*. These cases should be discussed with the practice accountant and agreement reached with the local Inspector of Taxes.

Depreciation

Depreciation of an asset is the means by which the cost of a capital investment is charged against income as an expense. Although a figure for depreciation is shown in the income and expenditure accounts, the actual tax benefit is determined through a tax claim for capital allowances (see next section).

There are various types of depreciation:

☐ *Straight line depreciation* – This is where an equal fraction of the cost of the asset is charged to depreciation in each year of its useful life, e.g. a commercial building may be depreciated over a 25 year period at 4% a year of its initial cost.

☐ *Accelerated depreciation* – This is where a fixed asset is depreciated more rapidly in the early part of its working life and more slowly later on, e.g. a motorcar will depreciate at 25% a year but on the reducing value.

☐ *Amortisation* is the process whereby intangible assets such as goodwill or leases are depreciated and charged against income over their useful life.

Capital allowances

As mentioned in Chapter 23, depreciation of capital assets is not allowable as a tax deductible expense. Instead the expenditure on such assets is set against tax by the system of *capital allowances* which are laid down by law.

The construction of most new buildings in an existing enterprise zone qualifies for a 10% initial allowance. Elsewhere, industrial and agricultural buildings attract a 4% a year writing down allowance but outside the enterprise zone these allowances will not be of help to small animal veterinary practices because retail shops, premises for the storage of retail items, showrooms and offices are regarded as non-industrial. However farm and equine veterinary practices may be able to claim the benefit of the writing down capital allowance if they have a building with an agricultural classification.

Expenditure on plant and machinery by small and medium sized enterprises (SMEs) qualify for a first year allowance of 40% for the tax year 1999/00 and later.

If there is a difference of opinion on a fair capital allowance for *plant* it can be worthwhile arranging an on-site meeting between the local

Inspector of Taxes and the practice accountant to agree an individual assessment.

Motorcars qualify for a 25% writing down allowance subject to an annual maximum of £3000. Veterinary instruments and equipment are regarded as plant and machinery and qualify for a 25% writing down allowance each year.

Short life assets such as veterinary instruments and equipment, which have a short life or a low value (say below £100) can be regarded as *replacement of tools* and are fully allowable as a business cost against profits in the first year. The costs of the leasing of capital equipment can also be claimed as a cost against profits each year

Major items of capital expenditure such as a new purpose-built veterinary hospital or a major extension to an existing premises will need to be funded by the introduction of fresh capital into the practice

Ongoing capital requirements to cover the replacement of cars, veterinary instruments and office equipment and the increasing cost in the replacement of existing assets should be funded out of a combination of retained profits and depreciation through the tax benefits of capital allowances. A percentage of annual turnover (say 2%) should be allotted each year to cover the cost of recurrent capital expenditure and be included in the forecast budget.

Timing of capital expenditure

A rolling three year budget should be agreed and revised each year for the ongoing capital expenditure with a list of priorities and an annual budget allocation. Capital allowances for motor cars and equipment can be claimed for the full year even if the purchase has taken place at the end of the financial year.

The decision on the timing of the annual budgeted items can be left until the second half of the year, and even until the last month, by which time an assessment can be made of the year's profitability and cash flow. If necessary the capital expenditure can always be postponed and carried over to the following year.

Appraisal of capital expenditure

In appraising future capital expenditure, you have to consider the time span over which the expenditure will be made, the extra revenue earned and the return on capital generated by the project.

Investment decisions on capital expenditure should be based on financial analysis of the investment proposal in order to reach a sound business judgment.

However, in veterinary practice it is accepted that there are many factors other than financial considerations which may play a major part in the decisions on future capital investment.

Capital investment analysis

Capital investment analysis is a qualitative financial assessment of capital projects and is of particular use when comparing the merits of different alternative capital projects. The making of sound assumptions and realistic forecasts is an integral part of the analysis – it is often said that in capital investment analysis 'the road to hell is paved with poor assumptions'.

The analysis will take into account all the relevant costs which are reflected in cash flows that change as a result of an investment decision but will not take into account *sunk* costs. These are costs already committed and are irrelevant for investment decisions. An example of a sunk cost would be the savings of cupboard or floor space following a change to automatic processing of radiographs.

There are a number of accounting methods used for capital investment:

Payback period
This is an assessment of the period of time which will elapse before the initial investment is recovered. The cash recovery period is the number of years for the cash coming in or the cost savings, to equal the cash going out.

In assessing the cash flows only the money *that rings up the tills* should be included, but the exception to this rule is when the tax benefit of depreciation is included.

A cash profile can be built up to calculate the payback period as shown in this example of a four year payback:

A practice decides to purchase a photocopier at a cost of £1500. This will save the expense of paying £400 a year to a local agency who has provided a photocopying service. There will be a tax benefit at the 25% rate for capital allowances on a 20% straight line depreciation over five years. The cost will be an annual payment of 10% interest on the reducing loan for the purchase of the photocopier.

Year capital	Cash in	Cash out	Net cash	Capital	Cumulative
	£	£	£	£	£
0	—	—	—	1500	1500
1	475	150	325		1175
2	475	118	357		818
3	475	82	393		425
4	475	43	432		0

Note: *Cash in* is £400 annual saving plus £75 capital allowance.
    Cash out is the cost of reducing interest payments.

Return on investment

The *return on investment* is the additional profit earned or the expected annual return as a percentage of the initial investment. It is calculated as:

$$\frac{\text{Expected annual return} \times 100\%}{\text{Invested capital}}$$

In the four year payback example this would be:

$$\frac{475 \times 100}{1500} = 31.7\%$$

Discounted cash flow

In making the detailed financial analysis, it is necessary to take into account the effect of the declining value of money. This is called *discounted cash flow*, and incorporates the principle of the time value of money.

Apart from inflation, the difference between the future value of money and its present value is the interest which could be accrued in the meantime. By deducting interest one can reduce future values to the equivalent present day values. The resulting figure is the discounted cash flow rate of return. Rates based on different interest rates can be obtained from tables (see Table 25.1 for example).

Table 25.1 Example of interest rate values.

Year received	Discounted cash flow rate (10%)	Value £
0	—	100
1	0.91	91
2	0.83	83
3	0.75	75
4	0.69	69
5	0.62	62

By using this principle of discounted cash flow it is possible to convert future costs to their net present values. This means that you can evaluate an investment proposition in terms of its present worth.

Chapter 26
The Ins and Outs of Cash Flow
Dixon Gunn

The concept of cash flow control is to ensure that money comes into the practice on a regular basis, with the appropriate gap between the 'in' and the 'out' to leave the reservoir (the bank account) at just the right level.

Depending on the circumstances of the practice, for example a newly established practice, or one in which there has been a recent change in partnership or even a major modernisation of property, the correct level for the bank account might be below zero – that is in overdraft. The maximum level of overdraft will have been agreed with the bank. Cash flow control should ensure that this level is not breached. It is no use waiting until some time after the end of the month, to find the bank statement presenting you with unwelcome figures, which are already two weeks out of date.

A very simple monitor can be run on a weekly basis by establishing on day one, the exact amount of money in the practice bank accounts and then each week adding to this sum the monies banked during the week, and subtracting the total value of all cheques written.

There are two aspects of cashflow. The first is knowing where you are at present, while controlling spending and maximising income. The second is the compilation of a cash flow projection to help to plan the practice year.

Petty cash

If, as is usually the case, the petty cash account is funded from cash received by the practice, which is diverted to the petty cash account rather than the bank, then this has no influence on the bank balance calculation. The petty cash account should only be used for very small purchases and should not be allowed to develop into a type of second practice bank, by holding a large amount of cash received in it. All sums added and their source, as well as all sums spent should be recorded so that the petty cash account balances every time.

Cash in hand, that is money actually on the practice premises in the form of bank notes or cheques, is inefficient money. It should be in a bank account, either saving interest or earning interest. This means putting all available money in the bank as frequently as possible. This has a hidden snag because banks charge businesses for all such transactions. Five inputs in one week will cost more than say two inputs in one week.

Bank charges

Bank charges have become a significant practice cost, but they are open to negotiation. It is important to know exactly how the bank is charging the practice and what it is doing for these charges. For example, many banks will allow a low percentage payment of interest on current accounts kept in the black, this interest being offset against charges. However, if the interest earned exceeds the charges, the bank does not credit you with the excess. It is therefore wrong to keep excess funds in a current account to counter charges.

In the established practice, with its cash flow moving smoothly, it is common to have 'cash rich' days at the bank and just before the end of the month 'cash poor' days at the bank. The bank will, on your instruction, monitor your current account on a daily basis and move funds to and from a deposit account or a business call account. In this way the current account is kept just positive and any extra money is 'on deposit' earning interest, until it is required.

The bank makes a charge for this service, as we charge in veterinary practice and hopefully, as in practice, the benefit to the client exceeds the costs. Recent developments in the banking world, including the demutualisation of building societies and the establishment of new banks has increased the opportunity of practices to select whom they wish to support. The route forward for each practice has not changed over the years but there is now a much greater variety of choice. Investigate the costs imposed on current account deposits and withdrawals, as well as the option to have a deposit account running in parallel with the current account without costs being imposed. The best solution may be to pay all practice monies into a deposit account and transfer a lump sum to cover current account payments as required.

As part of the cash flow control, it is important to know the best way to bank the money received and the only way to find out is to talk to the people you entrust with your cash. To be in a strong position to negotiate, it is essential to have a constant stream, or river, of cash coming in. The main sources are fees earned and medicines sold.

The value of having the account settled at the time cannot be overemphasised. Small animal practice is fortunate in being able to insist to a large degree on this arrangement. Depending on geographical area, social strata of clients and the attitude of the practice, small animal work can achieve from 60% to 99% of accounts settled at the time, with enormous benefits for cash flow. As an example, drugs dispensed and paid for by the client may not yet have been paid for by the practice.

The actual cost of raising a client account is considerable: a new name and address on the ledger or on the computer, an invoice produced, copied and posted, all for one small consultation.

Invoices

The farm client expects an account and in fairness, if the monthly invoice carries a large number of items, then the cost per item of maintaining that account is very much lower, but it is still there. In addition the cost of outstanding debts is real and varies with the cost of money. If the bank rate is 10%, then the cost of an outstanding debt is 1% to 1.2% per month, depending on the agreed overdraft rate. It is therefore critical for a practice running an accounts system to contain the outstanding debt. This is best monitored by the simple equation of:

$$\frac{\text{Outstanding debt} \times 365}{\text{Annual turnover minus cash at time}}$$

VAT is excluded from all the calculations and 'cash at time' is shorthand for all monies received at the time of provision of the service or the dispensing of drugs, whether it be in cash, by cheque or credit card. The answer in days is comparable year to year and an ideal to aim for is 45 days. This is rarely achieved and the greater the failure the greater the cost to the practice and the greater the pressure on cash flow.

One fact is very clear, the submission of full, easily read invoices within a day or two of the end of the month is most significant in achieving the required result, which is the payment of that invoice before the end of the current month.

Discounts for prompt payment usually have a greater effect than penalties for late payment. Those willing to risk a penalty are usually in cash flow turbulence themselves and are quite happy to use the practice as a further source of finance.

To help cash flow into the practice all personnel must keep up to date with their 'work invoices'. These invoices should be written at the time so that nothing is forgotten. 'Personnel' includes veterinary surgeons and support staff. General sales list products are frequently sold by support staff. Forgotten items, those not recorded on practice invoices, still constitute a serious loss of income and cash flow in many practices. Nobody wants to be guilty of this omission, and the way to overcome it is by adhering strictly to an agreed system.

Technology is helping with this problem. Small animal invoices are prepared on the computer in the consulting room or in the dispensary and printed at reception to wait for the departing client.

In the large animal and equine world hand held terminals are available so that the work done and drugs used and dispensed can be recorded against the client's name before the veterinary surgeon leaves the premises. The terminal is then downloaded into the practice computer accounts program on return to base. Even so, the only way to minimise the human error is to adhere strictly to the system of recording everything at the time.

Cash 'out'

Having maximised 'cash in' at as early a date as is possible, 'cash out' must be minimised and at as late a date as is possible. There are a number of rules to adhere to. The first is to consider carefully any discounts offered and to compare this with the cost of borrowing from the bank to pay the account if the practice has an overdraft. For example, a 5% discount for settlement by a given date is more than likely worth taking up even if the bank is charging you 20%. A £1000 account with a 5% discount becomes a £950 cheque paid out. £950 borrowed from the bank at 20%, will run 96 days before the interest payable is £50.

If there is no incentive to pay by a certain date, it is very wrong to put the account aside and pretend to forget it. Practices are recognised by those who supply them with goods and services in the same way as the practice recognises its own clients. The account should be paid as late as is appropriate but never so late as to damage the reputation of the practice. The practice may wish to return to the same source for future goods or services. If the provider is suspicious of reliability, the deal will be less advantageous.

Some outgoings are reinforced by law if made late. Income tax and VAT must be paid by the due dates or interest and penalties apply. These subjects are dealt with in other chapters.

It is helpful to recognise payments in four different categories. There are tax allowable payments, for example drugs purchased by the practice and salaries paid. There are capital sums to be paid out, for example purchase of a new car. This payment is not directly tax allowable, so timing of purchase must be considered. There are the statutory payments already mentioned, Inland Revenue payments (PAYE, self employed tax under Schedule D and National Insurance contributions) and VAT. These must be paid on time.

Finally there are the internal practice payments, partners' drawings, pension premiums and other personal expenses. If not controlled, this particular group can seriously upset cash flow. This is dealt with more fully in Chapter 14 Partners' Responsibilities.

The capital sums are paid out of taxed income. This means that £128 of net profit less tax at 22% will buy an article worth £100. As these items are usually large, e.g. a car or an X-ray set, forward planning is required, so that spending can be evened out over the year.

There is one particularly good time to purchase a capital item and that is just before the end of the practice financial year. As soon as an item is purchased a capital allowance can be set against the purchase price for tax purposes. As of 5 April 2000, first year allowances for purchases of equipment by small businesses has been set at 40%. Veterinary practices qualify as small businesses. This means that £1000 spent on a piece of veterinary equipment can claim £400 as a capital allowance and reduce taxable profits by the same amount. After the year of purchase the allowance reverts to 25% P.A.

Currently and up to 1 April 2002, expenditure on communication technology equipment, for example, practice computers, qualifies for a 100% first year allowance. The interpretation in a practice is that £5000 spent on a qualifying piece of equipment reduces net profits by £5000 and the tax bill by £2000. It is always best to seek professional advice on tax planning matters and to take an all round view. Beware of the tax tail wagging the financial dog. The recognition of such benefits as capital allowance have also to be carried forward in the cash flow projection as the write offs are not immediately available in terms of cash flow.

The vast majority of payments made by a practice are tax allowable and form part of the profit and loss account. From the cash flow point of view, careful housekeeping can even out the sums paid out each month. For example, four new tyres for a car can be held over to the first of the new month and their payment on the garage bill will not be due for a further seven weeks, on the 20th of the subsequent month.

Stock in hand

Purchase of drugs is likely to be one of the largest payments made each month. Most practices are overstocked with drugs, with the consequences of stock going out of date and money being tied up on the shelves to the detriment of cash flow. The cash has been sidetracked into a backwater. Stock level should be around 30 days measured by the formula:

$$\frac{\text{Stock in hand} \times 365}{\text{Annual drug purchase}}$$

As with outstanding debts, it costs 1% to 1.2% per month to keep stock on the shelf. The figure obviously varies with current interest rates (see Chapter 18).

Cash flow forecast

A cash flow forecast is a forecast of likely income received based on previous history and modified by budget figures, along with an expenditure plan taking care of necessary monthly payments, recognising the timing of statutory payments, forward planning of capital expenditure and controlling internal payments.

Preparing a cash flow forecast is a useful exercise for all practices, and it is essential for the new practice. An example is shown in Fig. 26.1.

Having thought about getting the cash in and paying debts at the appropriate time, a cash flow forecast simply adds these two parts together and forecasts the bank statement at the end of each month.

This exercise is the only practice monitoring exercise which includes VAT along with all other income and expenditure. This is because VAT is

Cashflow forecast commencing January 20XX				
	JAN	FEB	MAR	ETC
	£	£	£	£
Receipts				
Total cash received				
Capital introduced				
Total receipts A				
Payments				
Drug purchases				
Salaries				
V.S. inc Employers NIC				
Nurses inc Employers NIC				
Others inc Employers NIC				
Total salaries				
Establishment costs				
Rent				
Rates				
Insurance				
Heat & Light				
Maintenance				
Total establishment costs				
Overheads				
Carcase disposal				
Maintenance contracts				
Hire of equipment				
Postage & carriage				
Telephone				
Subscriptions				
Training				
Stationery				
Advertising				
Laboratory fees				

Overheads *(cont.)*				
Second opinion fees				
Insurance				
Accountancy				
Legal fees				
Laundry & cleaning				
Sundries				
Total overheads				
Vehicle & travel				
Motor expenses				
Leasing costs				
Hire purchase				
Insurance				
Total travel				
Finance				
Bank charges				
Bank interest				
Loan interest inc HP				
Leasing charges				
Credit card charges				
Total finance costs				
Other				
VAT payments				
Capital payments				
Partners' drawings				
Total other				
Total payments	B			
Net cash flow	A – B = C			
Opening bank balance	D	D	E	
Closing bank balance	D + C = E			

Fig. 26.1 Sample cash flow forecast

a positive or negative cash flow at the time, even though in terms of practice performance it is neutral at the end of the day. The practice pays Customs and Excise all VAT received, less all VAT paid, and the resultant effect on the practice is zero. But in cash flow terms, payments do not match each other precisely in time and will involve more than one month.

The forecast must set about predicting the month by month income received. Debtors are not included until they have paid.

From the income all monies to be paid out must be forecast and it is the actual sums paid out, not a proportion, because the payment will last a year. For example an insurance premium on property will fall due in say, January. The benefits of the policy will extend over twelve months and in writing a practice budget, it can be argued that in effect one twelfth of the total is paid each month. Not so for cash flow. The whole sum falls due in January.

Heat, light, telephones, etc., fall due once a quarter and like VAT are often paid in the month following the due date. So VAT due to the end of March is a cost in the April cash flow column.

Some costs must be estimated, for example the garage bill will depend on miles travelled, the drug bill will depend on how busy the practice is, whereas some can be precise. Wages of full time staff will be constant until the next wage award. Rents can be fixed for a number of years.

As in budgeting, some estimates have to be made, but in cash flow forecasting, never forget that the exact moment the money has to be paid out is the significant date.

Having deducted outflow from inflow will provide the next cash at bank figure and this is the starting point of the following month. The forecast should provide three things: proof that the financial position at the bank will steadily improve; when planned capital expenditure should take place (that is when funds will be available), and it might even indicate that an additional partners' drawing should be available in December, just in time to plan the skiing holiday.

Knowing where you are and where you are going to be is essential for the efficient practice.

Chapter 27

Management Accounts

Dixon Gunn

All businesses need to know about their own performance before anyone else does. Would any business want the bank manager or a major creditor such as the drug wholesaler to suggest that the practice may not be doing too well because the overdraft is climbing or payment of accounts is slipping? If an outsider points out a downturn before the partners know of it, then it could be suggested that the partners have failed in their duty.

Directors of limited companies have a legal obligation to care for their company and to know what is happening to it. Principals and partners have no such legal obligation but they have a moral obligation to care for their staff and the animals of their clients. Keeping track of practice performance is now an essential element of practice management. Fortunately it has never been easier to do so because of the often maligned computer which can produce information viewed simplistically as the old fashioned ledger printed out on the computer screen as a spreadsheet.

The major benefit of this is that with only a very small knowledge of algebra, the spreadsheet can be made to subtract, divide, transfer figures to other calculations etc. What is even better is that if a figure has been typed in error it can be corrected and all consequential changes because of this alteration will be carried out automatically.

Purpose of management accounts

Management accounts are a versatile tool, showing what the principal or partners want to know at the end of every month. They are accounts generated within the practice for the purpose of monitoring practice performance. They are not for external use; their purpose is up to date in house analysis.

Given that management accounts answer questions about the practice's performance, what are the questions to be asked? The first questions are simple, for example: 'What was the turnover for the month? What were the expenses for the month? What profit was left for the owners?'

The next question comes quickly to the enquiring mind: 'Why was turnover so low (bad) or so high (good); why were expenses so high (bad), low (good)?'

Explanations for the good or poor performance are required and then the question is: 'Is it always the same at this time of year?' Historical comparison is only possible if management accounts from previous years are available.

The final questions at this stage concern practice performance measured against what was hopefully anticipated – the budget. (See Chapter 24)

Budgets are nothing more than estimates of future performance. If you consider that things never work out as planned and so there is no point in having a budget, then you are staring into a black hole. It must be better to set budget targets for both income and expenditure and encourage all members of the practice to work towards these aims. The budget targets must be realistic.

Requirements of management accounts

Content

They should record every financial fact the principal, partners or practice manager may want to know. In terms of income, this might be fees earned and drugs sold in both small animal and equine work, (i.e. four items).

Greater detail is possible, for example fees earned on consultations, surgical work, laboratory work in small animal practice and the cost of pet foods and the value of pet food sales might be included. Similarly, on the cost side of the equation, management accounts might include details about the cost of running each assistant's car or the overtime paid to support staff each month. There is no limit to the range covered by management accounts, but to justify the investigation and the work of compilation, the answers must be of value to the practice.

The facts must be recorded under the correct headings. This means that income from whatever source must be capable of being allocated to its correct slot, for example farm visit fees, small animal drug sales and equine surgical procedures. Costs must also be correctly allocated, for example, carcase disposal, CPD courses, advertising, charitable gift and so on.

Ideally there should be no income left to be described as 'other' and no expenses left to be described as 'sundries'.

Period covered

Income for the month of January XXXX must relate to work done and drugs and other products sold during that month, whether paid for at the time or still outstanding at 1 February XXXX.

At the same time, monies received during January XXXX for work done and products sold in the previous December, or before, should *not* be included in the January income.

All costs incurred during January XXXX must be included. This means, in the case of the drug wholesaler's account, that the January account received by the practice around about 5 or 6 February is the sum to include for drug purchases, not the sum *paid* in January XXXX which actually represents the purchases in the previous December.

Other items cause more confusion. For example, if some painting and redecorating was carried out during January XXXX but no invoice has been received by 12 February, when management accounts for January are about to be produced what is the correct procedure? In this case, use the estimate or quotation given and adjust the February management accounts one month later by adding or subtracting the difference in the actual sum from the previous estimate.

The golden rule is 'only include income and expenditure which relate to the actual month'. However, this is complicated in the case of an annual payment in advance, for example professional indemnity insurance or property insurance. If the whole sum is payable in January is this a January expense or is it a monthly expense at one twelfth of the annual sum? Either treatment is acceptable as long as it is consistently applied. Charging one twelfth per month can be considered as more accurate in terms of recording practice expenses.

Completeness

Some items are easily forgotten, invariably costs; income is remembered, costs can be forgotten.

Direct debits and standing orders must be included. If there are monthly payments of regular amounts, these can be the first figure recorded for the new month. If they are variable, then reference to the bank statement is necessary. Bank charges and interest automatically claimed must be recorded upon receipt of bank statements.

Depreciation is another management accounting entry. The sophisticated practice will allocate depreciation on equipment and cars on a monthly basis. An effort should be made to do this. If this is not done, the basic method is to depreciate the value of equipment and motor vehicles as shown in the most recent accounts at the agreed practice rate per month.

Items which should not be included

There are three very important categories to consider here. The first is *capital expenditure* on, say, a new scanner or car. Capital expenditure is not part of the profit and loss account of the practice, and as such must not be included in management accounts recording profit and loss activities. By all means keep a separate record of capital expenditure and work out the monthly depreciation to be used in the management accounts.

Drawings should also be recorded on a separate system. They are not part of the practice management accounts. The bottom line of a practice profit and loss account is the net profit of the principal or partners. Whatever drawings the partners take out of these net profits during the year for personal living allowances, income tax, NI payments, pension payments and so on must come out of the bottom line net profits. Some practices allocate partners' salaries, but these are not salaries as for an employee. Once again these are drawings.

The third item is VAT, tax which the government has passed to the self-employed owners of a practice to implement on their behalf. Some items

are chargeable to VAT, many are not. The only clear way to record
practice performance is to exclude VAT from all recorded entries in the
management accounts. Management accounts should be a VAT free zone.
A separate VAT record is of course essential.

Setting up the system

Having thought through what the practice wants to know month by
month, the only starting point possible is to begin recording the facts from
the first day of the selected month. There will be no previous history to
compare with and probably no budget figures to aim at. It doesn't matter,
start recording practice activities month by month.

The first series of column titles are very simple. They are:

❏   Current month
❏   YTD

Current month is self explanatory, YTD is year to date. So, if the year
starts in January XXXX, YTD at the end of March XXXX represents the
sum of three months activity.

When the first year is completed there is a history to compare with and
for the progressive practice the basis of a budget. Suddenly the two
columns need to be extended and can then run over two pages of print-
out if required. The spreadsheet page can be as big as is required. The
column titles can be seen in Fig. 27.1, along with detailed titles for
income and expenditure in a mixed practice. Customise the list to fit your
practice.

A moving annual total (MAT) column which is in effect a year to date
figure representing the last 12 months at any one time can be included. For
example, when including March 2002 results in the MAT column, the
March 2001 results will drop out so that an annual total is always
available but is moving month by month.

For ease of comparison, each of the above columns should include
figures showing all income and expenses as a percentage of turnover (see
Fig. 27.2). The importance of this cannot be over emphasised; it helps the
busy principal or partner to read the management accounts quickly and
identify the out of line percentage result, for example, pet food sales down,
car costs up, advertising well up – why?

The two columns named VAR in Fig. 27.2 record the percentage variation between the actual figure and the budget figure, whether it be up or
down. Monthly variations from budget are common. For this reason the
year to date figures gain importance as the year goes on.

After six months the practice will have produced a half year set of
accounts within 2 weeks of the end of the period and it can immediately
compare these results with where it had hoped it would be.

Management accounts are designed to make it easy for those in control

INCOME
FEES
Small animal
Equine
Large animal
LVI (DAFS)
OVS
Any other fee income
TOTAL FEES

DRUG SALES
Small animal
Equine
Large animal
TOTAL DRUG SALES

OTHER INCOME

TOTAL INCOME

EXPENDITURE
Drug purchases

SALARIES
VS inc Employers NIC
Nurses inc Employers NIC
Others inc Employers NIC
TOTAL SALARIES

ESTABLISHMENT COSTS
Rent
Rates
Insurance
Heat & light
Maintenance
TOTAL ESTABLISHMENT COSTS

OVERHEADS
Carcase disposal
Maintenance contracts
Hire of equipment
Postage & carriage
Telephone
Subscriptions
Training
Stationery
Advertising
Laboratory fees
Second opinion fees
Insurance
Accountancy
Legal fees
Laundry & cleaning
Depreciation
Sundries
TOTAL OVERHEADS

VEHICLE & TRAVEL
Motor expenses
Leasing costs
Hire purchase
Depreciation
Insurance
Loss/profit on sale
TOTAL TRAVEL

FINANCE
Bank charges
Bank interest
Loan interest inc HP
Leasing charges
Credit card charges
Bad debts
TOTAL FINANCE

TOTAL EXPENSES

NET PROFIT

Fig. 27.1 Titles for analysis of income and expenditure in a mixed practice

Month				Last year			Year to date					YTD Last year		
Actual		Budget		Var.	Actual		Actual		Budget		Var.	Actual	
£	%	£	%	%	£	%	£	%	£	%	%	£	%

Fig. 27.2 Management accounts column titles

to see what is happening and it is then up to them to take steps to investigate variances or anomalies they do not understand.

The practice accountant should be given details of the practice management accounts after they have been set up so that the annual accounts can follow the same format. This will make interpretation of annual accounts easier and may help to reduce accountants' work and fees, as the practice can supply accurate information to their accountants in a useable form.

Interpretation

Good management accounts are easy to interpret. The first stage is to identify any figure which is out of line, both in respect of history and budget. Use of percentages aids this progress, but remember that a percentage decrease in, for example, equine fees might well be more than compensated for by a large increase in the percentage attributed to small animal fees. If the percentage is out of line look at the actual financial figures.

YTD figures increase in significance as the year runs on. The variance between YTD (budget) and YTD (actual) is a very important result which must be explained. The investigation will be assisted by comparison with peer groups parameters which can be provided by taking part in the various surveys of practice performance. Two costs are of particular importance to all practice:

❏ the cost of drugs and disposables as a percentage of turnover
❏ the cost of salaries and wages as a percentage of turnover.

Performance parameters should be measured both against internal results and external peer group results. There is no long term benefit in reducing the cost of staff by 0.5% year on year if the peer group is already 5% below the practice result.

Investigation

Occasionally a result will be thrown up that is not easy to explain. It might be an apparent failure to achieve the perceived mark up on drug sales or an unanticipated increase in support staff overtime payments. In these circumstances, an internal audit has to be conducted. This amounts to a detailed examination of what actually happened and a comparison made with what was expected.

The audit should explain the discrepancy. The next action is to refine the system to prevent the same discrepancy re-occurring.

Summary

Good management accounts enable the partners and practice manager to keep up to date with practice performance. In addition, in to-day's changing practice structure, the management accounts can be the biggest aid the practice manager has in discussing and advising the owner(s) on practice performance.

Chapter 28
Construction of a Fee

Dixon Gunn

The construction of the fee you charge your clients for carrying out veterinary work on their behalf should have a logical basis. It is important in our modern society that this be so, because we are more likely now than ever before to be questioned on our fees or asked to quote a fee in advance for a routine procedure. We should be able to justify our response.

'Fees' refer to payment for the provision of a service whether it be a clinical examination, a surgical intervention or advice given without 'hands-on' contact. Fees do not include the sale of veterinary medicines as a part of, or in parallel to, the provision of a service. The sale of medicines should be seen as a separate department of the practice, where it is essential to sell the medicines at a price which ensures that the cost price, plus the storage costs and the losses due to 'out of dates', broken bottles and 'left on shelf' items, are recovered as well as a profit on the exercise. A dispensing fee, if charged, is a fee for providing the service and is not linked to the value of the commodity.

Earning time

All the costs of the practice other than those related to medicines have to be recovered by the fees in the fee earning time available in each day.

Fee earning time is to some extent outside our control, as we are requested to carry out services on a very *ad hoc* basis, but in the established practice the average day will show average results and this means that out of an approximately nine hour working day, we will be fee earning for only some four to seven hours. This excludes driving time which is of great significance in large animal and equine work.

The gap between four hours chargeable time (farm work) and seven hours chargeable time (small animal work) highlights the problem of how to charge for miles driven. If a standard LVI type mileage fee is charged, this covers nothing more than the running and maintenance costs of the vehicle. In this situation all other costs of the practice must be recovered from work chargeable hours.

The number of fee earning hours is critical because when multiplied by the number of working days in the year it provides us with the total number of hours for which we can charge our clients in a year. If we know how much we need to earn for the practice (exclusive of VAT) in a year then it is simple to determine what our hourly rate must be.

Costs

What we need to earn for our practice can be forecast year to year with some degree of accuracy, but it will only be accurate if all the costs, obvious and less obvious, are added in. Examples of obvious costs are as follows.

❑ *Salaries* of veterinary staff, support staff and part-time help. Remember to include employer's National Insurance contributions.
❑ *Motoring costs:* garage bills, road fund tax, car insurance as well as depreciation on the vehicle and interest on the capital invested in this piece of practice equipment. Depreciation and interest on capital invested should perhaps be classified as less obvious costs; whichever, they are real costs of the practice. These are the costs which should be recovered in the mileage charge.
❑ *Establishment costs* which include rent, rates, water rates, building and contents insurance, heating and lighting as well as maintenance of the premises.
❑ *Other overhead costs.* It is important not to forget the real cost of providing the service so a brief list of items to remember is as follows:
   machine rentals
   postage, packing and carriage
   telephone
   laboratory fees
   carcase disposal
   accountancy, legal and consultancy fees
   interest
   bank charges
   subscriptions
   course expenses
   laundry and cleaning
   stationery
   bad debts written off
   depreciation of instruments and equipment
   sundries

Sundries have to include all the odd items and it is essential to record all expenses. For accounting purposes and VAT purposes keep all receipts of payments made.

The less obvious costs which are equally important in that they must be recovered in the fees the practice charges if the business is to continue to thrive, are sometimes called *notional* costs. They are called *notional* because they are not actually paid month by month but they are still real in a business sense.

The first cost to consider is the capital invested in the practice properties. Are you just to invest this money without a return on the capital or indeed without an income by way of fees charged to enable you to plan development, upkeep and repair of the practice properties? The combined return for investment and future planning should bring in at least 10% per annum of current cost of replacing buildings. There is other capital involved in the practice excluding cars and property already taken into account, and again this should show a return of, say, 2% over base rate in a properly run business.

Counting through the costs listed to date, it will be rapidly noted that so far there is no salary or net profit for the self-employed owner or partner. This should not be ignored until the end of the year nor should it be put in at a ridiculous figure. About $1\frac{1}{2}$ times an assistant's salary, including employer's National Insurance contribution, is a reasonable salary for a partner and allows some payment into a pension policy.

The final and quite legitimate cost to build in is a profit margin over and above everything else. It acts as a buffer if costs escalate or work diminishes. The margin could be 10% of the other costs.

Calculation of hourly fee

Having summed all of these costs, the resultant figure is the sum you have to recover in fees over a year (excluding VAT and all drug and other product sales).

The sum required in the year 2000 can be suggested as £115 000 per veterinary surgeon in a purely small animal practice and £93 000 per veterinary surgeon in a purely large animal practice. Note that these figures exclude the cost of travel which is presumed to be recovered via mileage charges.

The annual fee required is reduced to an hourly fee by dividing the toal sum by the work chargeable hours per year. Most practices will not be aware of this figure for their practice. To assist, it can be suggested that a full time equivalent veterinary surgeon in small animal practice could record some 1566 work chargeable hours a year and a colleague in large animal practice some 1166 work chargeable hours annually. Mixed practice falls between the two, depending on the mix of work.

The use of these figures suggests an hourly fee of £73 in small animal practice and £80 per hour in large animal practice.

These fees are not achieved in practice and the necessary support of the shortfall is covered by profit earned on the sale of medicines and ancillaries. Dependence on such support is not secure and practices should make every effort to cover the costs of providing their services from the fees earned.

Notional costs as detailed above are real and failure to recover these costs diminishes the ability of the practice to develop and improve its facilities and its service to the client.

Fee per job

Translating the required hourly fee into a job fee is simple. A ten minute consultation is one sixth of an hourly fee, a lame cow taking 20 minutes of time is one third of an hour and so on.

Surgery often confuses people by seeming to be priced at a higher rate, but consider not only the actual theatre time, but the admission time, in-hospital time, preparation time, discharge time and suture-out time. This doubles the actual theatre time which is usually the only time people remember.

Similarly, out of hours consultations and visits actually take very much longer than routine work and as such justify a higher fee.

Finally, if the fee is not right, by which I mean too low, then the reward for the people involved will be too low and even more importantly the practice will not thrive, develop and improve its service to the animals under its care.

Chapter 29

Securing Income

Dixon Gunn

A subheading for this chapter might be 'debt collecting' but if this is necessary it is already too late. The aim is to not have debts, but to have all those clients running accounts settling within the agreed time scale.

Practice income falls into two major groups, payment at the time and payment on receipt of an account.

Payment at the time

The value of cash at the time cannot be overstated. There is money in the bank supporting the practice account immediately and no need to post an invoice, a follow up statement or a reminder, all of which cost time and money. In addition the accounts system in the practice can be much simpler and of course if the sum owed is paid at the time there is no possibility of it developing into a bad debt.

How then to get clients to pay at the time? This has to start with a decision by the practice on its approach to the subject and everyone involved has to know of this approach. It can be as slack as 'ask the client to pay and if they say no, send them an account', or it can be 'we will not treat the animal or sell the product unless they pay at the time' which is impossible to impose because the animal has been treated before the debate on payment takes place.

The practice must set its own rules and in small animal work this should be aimed at getting everyone to pay at the time and making it difficult not to pay. This can start before the consultation with the receptionist asking politely how the client would like to pay, by cash, by cheque or by credit card? Care must be taken in the selection of cards accepted. Rates of interest vary as does the delay before the money reaches the practice bank. These costs should be built into the fee structure of the practice.

If the client looks puzzled or irritated at being asked about payment prior to being seen, then a smiled apology at the same time as directing the client's attention to the practice policy clearly stated in a notice saying: 'Clients are requested to pay for all services and medicines at the time. Credit cannot be given without prior arrangement.' If the client then immediately asks for credit, at least the practice has been forewarned. This policy notice should be displayed everywhere that clients might debate whether or not to pay. This can include a reception point for farmers and/ or horse owners in a mixed practice.

The basis is that credit cannot be given without prior agreement. If such agreement is requested by a client and given by the practice, then at that point the practice should explain its terms of trading. This is discussed under the heading Account clients below.

Invoice production

To make it easy for clients to pay at the time a quick and efficient method of producing an invoice has to be available. The small animal method of choice is to have a computer system linking together consulting rooms, dispensary and front desk. The veterinary surgeon or a nurse raises the invoice in the consulting room or dispensary, with the items being automatically priced by computer code. The invoice should be detailed with each procedure identified, for example, laboratory tests and X-rays. Each medicine should be named and separately priced. The client should be able to see and understand what the pet has received. The client returns to the front desk where the detailed invoice is printed out in front of the client, passed over for examination and agreement, and payment made before the dispensed medicines are handed over. The invoice should be receipted with a practice stamp as proof of payment. This protects both the client and the practice.

The same system can be used in a practice with large PML sales. The farmer requests the medicines, is directed to the pick up point where the invoice is produced prior to handing over the drugs. Telephone orders are collected from the same point, using the same method if it is a cash sale. Even with this type of efficient system difficulties will arise. The client has agreed to pay cash and then 'Oh dear, purse or wallet has been left at home'. The carefully prepared invoice is still printed, possibly marked to be paid and if possible only enough medicine or tablets for 24 hours are dispensed with the request that the client returns next day to collect the rest of the treatment and pay the invoice.

Some still get away. Good client records annotated accordingly should mean that non-payers only manage this once, as he or she can be challenged on the outstanding sum prior to being seen or allowed to make a purchase on a subsequent visit to the practice. Other than sending a statement and a written demand for the outstanding sum, it is rarely worth spending time and money attempting to collect relatively small sums. It is better to perfect the system of identifying the non-payers and refusing them all but acute emergency first aid in the name of animal welfare.

Account clients

Every account client should have made an agreement with the practice at the time of setting up an account. In the main these will be farmers, riding schools, studs, boarding kennels, dog breeders and the like. These are often large accounts with a number of visits per month made to the establishment.

The higher risk accounts are the single horse owner, the hobby farmer and the small animal owner with many pets and too little income.

Terms of trade

Before any client receives any agreement to pay on account, the terms of trade should be clearly explained. These should be printed out and a copy given to each client. The terms will vary with the practice philosophy but might cover all or some of the following points.

(1) Invoices will be raised on every occasion on which a sale of services or medicines is made.
(2a) A statement with invoice copies will be sent within four working days of the end of each calendar month, *or*
(2b) A statement detailing these invoices will be sent within four working days of the end of each calendar month.
(3) A discount of 5% may be deducted for payment by the 20th of the month.
(4) A surcharge of 5% will be added if the statement has to be resubmitted in the following month.
(5) An interest charge of 2% per month will be added to all accounts outstanding at the end of the second month.
(6) Any complaint regarding sums billed must be notified to the practice within fourteen days of receiving the account.

Submission of accounts

Options (2a) and (2b) above are included for the following reason. The invoice should be produced at the point of sale, that is on the farm, at the stable or in the surgery. If this routine is strictly adhered to, then the chance of forgetting to book items is lessened but not eliminated. Such an on the spot production usually means that the invoice will be handwritten and very often in shorthand as well.

For clarity this should be translated onto the statement in some detail giving invoice number, date, veterinary surgeon initials and individual lines for services provided and drugs dispensed so that each cost can be identified. In this case the full statement would be submitted but the copy invoices would not. If the statement merely records the invoice number, then the detailed invoice should be included with the statement, unless it has already been provided at point of sale.

As systems improve, hand held terminals will be more widely used. The veterinary surgeon on the farm will key in the relevant details and on return to the surgery will download the information straight into the accounts program on the computer.

The end of month statement is made up day by day and will be available for printing and dispatch at 9.00 AM on the first working day of the month. That can only happen if everyone has compiled, produced and then downloaded all their invoices. The fact that a practice does not send out accounts until the 14th of the month or later, sends out a huge delay message to clients. The human mind says: they were slow sending the bill, so I can be slow paying. Equally, a clearly worded statement produced very shortly after the month end says 'We are accurate and efficient' and the recipient responds by saying 'That's true, I must be seen to be the same and pay promptly'.

What of the slow payers? If the practice is using a discount or surcharge system these must be imposed. Do not allow discount to be taken after the due date and do not accept late payment without the surcharge. Refer the client to the terms of trading they agreed to. There must also be an agreed system for chasing outstanding accounts. Possible action might include the following.

(1) A note or sticker on the second statement pointing out that the previous month's account is overdue.
(2) A personal letter demanding payment one month after first sub-mission. A request to contact and discuss can offer a way out to the client at this point.
(3) Referral to a debt collector, solicitor, small claims court, etc., if still unpaid one month later. That is if, for example, January's work, billed in February, is still not paid for by the end of April.

Some practitioners like to pay a personal visit to the debtor and confront him or her. Some veterinary surgeons find this intimidating. The method of debt collecting is a personal decision.

Professional debt collectors either charge a fee whether or not they are successful or a percentage of what they recover. Discuss their methods and likely costs before instructing them. The same holds good for a solicitor. Discuss how they approach the subject. Do they have a debt collection department within their practice and what will the likely costs be?

Going to court can be time consuming if undertaken personally and can be expensive if the practice buys its representation. Even though the sums are likely to be much larger than the small animal debt, the costs are also likely to be larger and once again a balance has to be struck if a Pyrrhic victory is to be avoided. It is perhaps financially sounder to write the client off as well as the bill and no doubt neighbouring practices could be made aware of your decision.

Securing income and avoiding debtors is essential to the well being of the practice.

Chapter 30
Buying a Property
John Gripper

Buying your first house or practice property is probably the most important financial investment you will make in your lifetime. The rise in house prices, over the years, has meant that the average veterinary surgeon in private practice is more likely to have increased his personal capital from his investment in residential and commercial property than from any growth in the business capital value of his practice.

There is a considerable variation of property prices around the country with prices in the south of England as much as twice as high as prices in the midlands and the north, but the pattern of house prices is constantly changing according to the growth of motorways and other local factors.

In view of the value of the investment you are making, as well as the personal commitment involved, professional financial advice should always be sought.

Planning permission

If you wish your property to be used as a veterinary surgery, and there is no existing planning permission then you will need to apply to the local authority. Any offer to purchase the property must be made conditional subject to receiving planning approval under the Town and Country Planning Act.

Your first step is to make a visit to the planning authority and discuss your proposed application with the planning officer. His main concern will be the possible nuisance to nearby residents from noise, smell and also inconvenience from additional car parking.

You should then go and talk to the immediate neighbours to put their minds at rest that your hospitalisation areas will be soundproof and your surgery will be hygienic with no unpleasant smells. Explain that your appointment system will mean that there will only be limited need for extra car parking.

Find out which local councillors sit on the planning committee and invite one or two of them (especially the pet owners) round to see the premises. Explain the need for a veterinary surgery in that area and your real concern to see that all pet animals receive proper skilled treatment and suggest that it is their public duty to support your application which will be bringing a necessary amenity to the area.

Your planning application will be advertised in the local paper which will provide the opportunity for local objections. Your planning permission may be granted subject to restrictions such as times of surgery hours, provision of sufficient own parking spaces, no boarding kennels and a ban on keeping animals overnight.

Whilst a restriction for no boarding and the keeping of animals overnight may be acceptable for the lock up branch surgery, it is essential that for the main surgery you establish that animals can be kept in for hospitalisation and emergency treatments such as post-operative care or road accidents.

Mortgages

It is possible to obtain a mortgage for up to 95% of the purchase price or valuation, whichever is the lower. However if the mortgage is higher than 75% of the value of the property then you may have to pay a mortgage indemnity guarantee policy, and the premium for this could be 4% of the amount advanced in excess of the 75% figure. This policy protects the lender, not you, if your home is repossessed.

The amount you can borrow may be as high as 3.25 × your gross annual income or for joint applicants, either 2.5 × joint income, or 3 × main income, plus that of your partner.

The above figures are only guidelines and in an extremely competitive mortgage market, some lenders are offering mortgages at higher income multipliers. Do however beware of overextending yourself with high mortgage repayments – these can become a major problem if interest rates rise significantly or if income is reduced because of changes in your personal circumstances, such as redundancy or pregnancy.

It is now possible to take out an insurance policy which will pay your monthly mortgage instalments if you are absent from work because of sickness, accident, unemployment or redundancy. These policies should only be viewed as a stop gap, as payment of benefits is normally restricted to a two year period, after an initial deferred period when no benefit is payable. Many people may elect to take out these policies commonly offered by banks and building societies and then top them up with a personal policy which would provide a source of permanent income in the event of serious illness or disability, when the mortgage insurance policy stops paying.

There is a wide variety of mortgages available, but these tend to fall into two distinct categories: *repayment* or *interest only* mortgages.

Under each arrangement, it is again possible to arrange a flexible (variable) rate of interest, or a mortgage offering a discount over a set period on normal variable or fixed rates.

Repayment mortgage
This is the traditional method whereby both the capital and interest are repaid over an agreed period. The interest rate can be fixed or variable.

It is important however to remember that in the early years, the majority of the monthly payments made will be interest so if a property move is made in the early years, little capital will have been repaid. This type of mortgage payment may therefore be more beneficial for those who are likely to stay in the property for some time.

Interest only mortgage

With an interest only mortgage, only interest payments are made to the lender each month and the capital is repaid at some time in the future from savings policies effected to run alongside the mortgage.

These savings policies may be selected to suit individual circumstances, but may be:

◻ *Endowment*: full or low cost
◻ *Pension*
◻ *Regular savings plans*: unit or investment trusts, or personal equity plans (PEPs).

In each case, whether electing for a repayment or interest only loan, it is essential that life cover is taken out to repay the debt in the event of death, during the mortgage term. For those who are self employed (or in non pensionable employment) this can be arranged with tax relief against the premiums payable.

This type of policy is known as *term assurance* (i.e. life cover only for a specified period) and may be arranged on a level or reducing basis.

The various means of accumulating capital to repay the lender may be:

Endowment mortgages

Only the interest and policy premium is paid on this type of mortgage, with the capital being repaid by the endowment policy when it matures at a predetermined age. The additional cost of the endowment premium is no longer tax allowable.

There may be a surplus of cash when the policy matures which is paid as a lump sum but this will depend on the investment performance and the bonuses allotted to the policy by the insurance company. The low cost endowment policies will not perform as well as the traditional endowment policies but both provide you with life cover.

Early surrender of endowment polices will attract heavy penalties. Some sales of unsuitable endowment policies have been motivated by the sales commission generated. The returns of some endowment policies have been disappointing in recent years, with a requirement for additional premiums to ensure adequate capital on maturity, as a result of which this type of policy is going out of favour. However an endowment with a good quality insurance company can still produce excellent returns over the years.

Pension mortgages

Only the interest on the loan and the pension premium is payable. The capital is repaid out of the tax free capital sum which is available when the personal pension policy matures. The pension premium is eligible for income tax relief at your highest tax rate which makes this form of mortgage very tax efficient.

Commercial mortgage loans

All the high street banks offer commercial mortgages. These can be arranged at fixed or variable interest rates and an endowment linked option is available.

A capital holiday for up to two years may be arranged at the outset of the repayment mortgage. A negotiation or arrangement fee will be charged. The interest paid on a business mortgage or loan is allowed as an expense against the practice.

Negative equity

Negative equity arises where the property is worth less than the value of the mortgage and the owner cannot afford to sell. This was brought about when home-owners bought overvalued houses between 1988 and 1992 with very large mortgages, and it has resulted in families being unable to move and in some cases losing their houses through repossession. Over the years the mortgage repayments will gradually reduce negative equity and house prices will start to rise again.

Valuation and surveys

You have a choice of three different types of survey and valuation according to your needs and the depth of your pocket.

Full structural survey

This is a detailed investigation into all the accessible parts of the property and should be undertaken by a qualified chartered surveyor. This survey will provide a comprehensive description of the structure of the property and a full list of the major and minor defects, plus an indication of the cost of repairs. The fee for a survey of this sort should be negotiated in advance.

Home buyer's survey and valuation report

This will be prepared on a standard form by the Incorporated Society of Valuers and Auctioneers (ISVA) or the Royal Institution of Chartered Surveyors (RICS) and will provide the purchaser with a concise and readable account of the general condition of the property, identifying general repairs and providing an assessment of its open market value.

This standard survey is acceptable for mortgage purposes and the fees should be agreed in advance. It will not be as comprehensive as a full structural survey which is recommended for larger properties (ten rooms or more than three storeys) or older properties (over 100 years old).

Report and mortgage valuation

This is a professional valuation to assess the suitability of the property as security for the mortgage or loan required. The inspection of the property will be very limited in its scope and no responsibility will be taken should major defects show up at a later date.

This type of valuation will be required by a bank or a building society before agreeing to a mortgage or a loan. There is a standard fee for a valuation report and you should always insist on receiving a copy of the report.

Estate agents

Under the Estate Agents Act 1979 anybody without qualifications or experience can set up as an estate agent. It is advisable to only deal with estate agents who are members of one of the recognised professional bodies, i.e. Royal Institution of Chartered Surveyors or the Incorporated Society of Valuers and Auctioneers who require their members to pass examinations. The National Association of Estate Agents demands evidence of three years trading before allowing an application for membership.

In the housing boom of the late 1980s most of the established firms were taken over by banks, building societies and insurance companies but this proved to be a disastrous investment and the majority of them are now back in private ownership.

Beware of financial institutions who wish to sell you a package of insurance and mortgage as they are usually 'tied' agents rather than independent and you may finish up with an unsuitable or more expensive policy than you require.

Stamp duty

This is a tax charged on the documents by which certain types of property are transferred to new owners. The current stamp duty rates for year 2000/01 are

£60 000–£250 000	1%
£250 000–£500 000	2.5%
£500 000 and over	3.5%

The rate of duty is assessed by reference to the aggregate amount payable on stampable items which include property, goodwill and permanent fixtures which cannot lawfully be separated from the property. Non-stampable items include virtually all items of plant and machinery and movable chattels including stock, drugs etc.

Contracts of sale

Legislation has ended the legal monopoly on conveyancing which was held by solicitors, and the necessary property searches and other paper-work can now be carried out by a licensed conveyancer. My advice is to always use a solicitor.

In Scotland a written offer to buy a property is made through a solicitor, and once accepted both parties are legally bound. If you buy a property at auction in England the conditions of sale are usually an immediate 10% deposit with completion in 28 days.

Under present legislation in England a verbal agreement is not binding in law until written contracts have been signed by both parties and exchanged; this allows a seller to back out of a property deal before contracts are exchanged and accept a higher offer – this is called *gazumping*.

Gazumping is a frustrating problem for the purchaser and can run up wasted costs for legal work and valuations. It flourishes at times of property shortages and rapidly rising house prices and is practised by greedy owners encouraged by unprofessional estate agents whose sales commission is based on the selling price.

A buyer can also change his mind and pull out of the deal which can cause considerable problems particularly if there is a chain of other people all waiting to buy and sell. *Reverse gazumping* is when the buyer threatens to back out at the last minute unless the price is lowered.

Once contracts have been exchanged the purchase is legally binding and a completion date is arranged. A 10% deposit is paid on exchange with the balance due on completion. The new owner becomes respon-sible for the insurance of the building as soon as contracts have been exchanged.

There is a clear case for a change in the conveyancing law in England to adopt a better system, in which once a written offer between buyer and seller is accepted then it becomes legally binding on both parties.

Pre-contract agreements between buyer and seller are now binding in law. For a period of usually two weeks, a seller promises not to negotiate with anyone else once a sale has been agreed.

In order to speed up the conveyancing of property in England and Wales, the government has proposed a scheme whereby the vendor obtains, at his expense, the property valuation and carries out the neces-sary searches.

Summary

Even in times of rapidly rising house prices it is unlikely that the full costs of buying and selling will be recouped if you have to resell within a year. These costs include legal fees, stamp duties, mortgage and insurance costs, and necessary repairs and decoration in a new house and have been estimated to represent about 10% of the property value.

When there is a stagnant housing market then the attractions of house purchase are much reduced. If you only plan to live in the area for a few years then rental of a property may be a preferred option.

While a newly qualified assistant should be considering the purchase of a house as soon as practicable to get a foot on the housing ladder, he should beware all the costs and hazards of house purchase such as contract races, gazumping, chains, bridging loans and unprofessional estate agents.

Chapter 31

A Tax on Income

Dixon Gunn

Everybody who makes a profit from providing a service or selling a product is liable to pay tax on this income. There are certain minimum levels below which nil tax is payable, but that income is still involved in the calculation of total tax payable.

As a profession we are divided into employed persons, who are qualified veterinary surgeons working for a practice or other organisations, and self-employed persons, who are principals or partners of a practice, or independent consultants. As an aside, we must also include directors, who are classified as employees of the company they serve.

There are considerable differences in the way in which employees are taxed on their income compared with the way in which self-employed persons pay their tax.

Employees

In Chapter 33 National Insurance and PAYE are discussed in terms of the duties of the employer. However, the employee must also take care of him or herself.

Each employee is given a tax code which determines how much tax is deducted from gross salary. The higher the code, the lower the deduction, so it is to the employee's benefit to maximise any legitimate claims. Subscriptions to professional societies, if paid personally, may qualify for relief. For example RCVS and BVA subscriptions qualify.

Unfortunately there is no tax allowance on premiums paid on life assurance policies taken out after 14 March 1984. For those holding policies taken out before this date the rate of relief is 12.5% of the premiums paid. From April 2001 *stakeholder pensions* are available. These are aimed at both employees and the self-employed to encourage them to augment their state pension by self investment.

Of more significance to the employee is the potential for investing in a personal pension plan, either outside the current government scheme or as an additional payment. Sums paid for personal pensions, within maximum limits which are generous, are paid free of tax. This means that each £100 of income paid into a pension fund is not taxed before payment, up to the statutory limits.

Employees in veterinary practice will often be supplied with a car, accommodation and the use of a telephone. Although all part of their employment, there are financial advantages in receiving these benefits as part of their appointment. Employers must complete a form known as a

P11D for each employee earning more than £8500. This figure of £8500 applies after adding the value of the benefits to the gross salary. This means that every full-time assistant in veterinary practice will exceed the limit. The effect of this is that the employee will be taxed on the benefits the Inland Revenue perceive to have been received. Although this aggravates both employees and employers, the perceived benefits may not be as punitive as the employee would find them to be if asked to provide the facility for him or herself.

As an example, the most commonly provided benefit is a practice car. The current method of assessment is first based on the list price of the car when first registered and the maximum benefit in kind is 35% of this list price for cars driven for less than 2,500 business miles p.a. This percentage drops to 25% for cars driven between 2,500 and 18,000 business miles p.a. and to 15% for cars driven in excess of 18,000 business miles p.a.

Each of the above percentages is reduced by one quarter if the car is at least four years old at the end of the tax year. In addition there are fuel scale charges running from £1,700 to £3,200 p.a. in year 2000/01 depending on engine capacity.

The net result of this is that, in 2000/01, the benefit in kind of having the private use of a car and free fuel, if the car is less than four years old, has an engine capacity of less than 2000 cc, has a list price of £10,000 and is driven between 2,500 and 18,000 business miles p.a., is £4,670. This is the sum on which income tax will be charged.

From April 2002 the whole system changes. Discounts for the number of business miles driven and the age of the car will be discontinued. The tax charge will be based on a percentage of the list price of the car graduated according to the level of the car's carbon dioxide emissions. The range runs from 15% to 35% of list price.

Self-employed

The move from employee status to self-employed can be stressful in that a tax demand appears to be forever hovering behind the shoulder of the veterinary surgeon who has just made the change. This is not so as the rules are very different.

The move to partnership and self-employment brings with it the need to conceive a completely different approach to 'take home pay'. The employee knows that what he takes home is his. The partner must recognise that what he takes home is only a payment on account of projected profits at the end of the year. If these profits exist at the end of the year then the drawings taken are recognised by Inland Revenue as pre-tax payments and income tax is taken out of the remainder of the profits. So even though the system is looser, just as much planning must be put in, if the practice is not to become an Inland Revenue debtor.

The allowances dealt with under 'employees' hold good for the self-employed. Payments for professional subscriptions and the like are normally paid by the practice and do not need to be claimed on a personal basis.

A practice may claim the costs of sending a partner or an employee to a continuing professional development (CPD) course. As current legislation stands an employee paying for himself to attend a CPD course cannot easily put this expense against taxable income. CPD for employees should be supported financially by the practices employing them.

After all claims on income are agreed, the partnership is left with a figure called 'net profit' and it is on this figure that their personal tax will be based. There is, however, an important variation to this figure before it appears as the taxable income of the practice. The variation is that depreciation as shown in the 'profit and loss account' is only for internal practice information. Depreciation, however represented, is not allowable for tax purposes and the sum allowed for depreciation in the accounts is added back to net profit, to be replaced later by a figure known as capital allowances, determined by rules laid down by Inland Revenue.

One of the major allowances that can be taken up is an investment in personal pension plans and as an extension of this, personal life insurance. Life insurance taken out under section 620 of the Income and Corporation Taxes Act 1988 allows a self-employed person to use a proportion of tax allowable premiums to pay for life insurance and receive full tax allowance on the premiums. If partners wish to insure their lives in trust for each other this is the best method of achieving this aim.

The major difference between being employed and being self-employed is that the self-employed only have to pay tax twice a year instead of every time they receive a pay cheque.

A practice may select any date as its personal end of year date. The calculation of tax payable is based on what is called *current year basis*. This means that a practice with an end of year date of 30 April will be assessed for the 2000/01 tax year on its profits for the practice year ending on April 30 2000, i.e. the practice year ending within the national financial year.

The tax is paid in two instalments, the first by January 31 within the current tax year and the second by July 31, after the end of the year of assessment. The instalments are usually half of the previous year's liability. Any under- or overpayment is corrected when actual figures become available.

Partners are assessed separately and are no longer jointly and severably liable for the total tax to be paid by the partnership.

Start up

When a new practice starts up profits are taxed in the following way.

In the first year, tax is assessed by reference to profits actually earned during the financial year from start up to the following 5 April. For example, a practice starting on 6 October will have traded for six months by 5 April following. The practice would normally draw up accounts to the following 5 October, one year after start up. The first year assessment will be 50% of this first year's profit representing the six months of trading to the previous 5 April.

The second year's assessment will normally be based on the profits of the first full year of trading to 5 October, one year after start up.

The third year of assessment is on the current year basis.

Cessation

When a partner retires or a business closes down, the individual assessment is based on the profits on the current year basis plus the profits to the date of retirement. For example, a partner retires on October 31 2002. The annual practice accounts are made up to 30 April each year. The retiring partner will be assessed on his share of profits to 30 April 2002 and in addition on his share of profits to 31 October 2002, the date of his retirement. Depending on the history of tax payments by the practice, he may be entitled to 'overlap relief' linked to his introduction as a partner.

Chapter 32

Value Added Tax

John Gripper

Value added tax was introduced in the UK on 1 April 1973 and is administered by Customs and Excise. Goods or services supplied by a veterinary surgeon as a registered trader are *outputs* and VAT is added at the standard rate.

The purchases made by the veterinary surgeon of goods and services for the purpose of his business are *inputs* and the input tax may be reclaimed from Customs and Excise.

Registration

A trader is liable for registration if at the end of any month the value of taxable supplies for the last twelve months exceeds the annual threshold of £52 000 a year. This is the current 2000/01 figure and is usually adjusted upwards by the Chancellor at each Budget.

A person whose taxable income is below the turnover limit may make an application for voluntary registration and this will allow the VAT on inputs to be reclaimed, but VAT will have to be charged on outputs as well.

When you start up a new practice it is advisable to seek registration in advance prior to making taxable supplies, so that you can claim back the VAT on your start-up costs, i.e. instruments and equipment, legal and professional fees, drugs, printing and motoring expenses, etc. Your application should be made on form VAT 1 and you will have to make an estimate of your expected taxable turnover. You would be advised to make an estimated figure which is above the minimum registration level.

Once you are a registered trader you will need to add VAT at the standard rate of 17.5% to all your fees and sale of drugs. When VAT was first introduced the client was often quoted a price plus VAT but now most practices will quote a VAT inclusive price to members of the public. A client who is registered for VAT, for example farmers, can claim back the VAT that you charge them and will need a taxable invoice which includes your VAT registration number.

VAT records

A registered trader must keep adequate records for at least six years. This VAT account must show the total inputs, total outputs and the tax invoices that have been issued and received with the VAT charged on them.

Where a taxable person has failed to make the required returns or to keep the proper records he is liable for a penalty and the Customs and Excise may make an assessment of the VAT due and the trader will have to pay that assessment.

VAT returns

A VAT return (Form VAT 100) to Customs and Excise must be made within one month of the end of the standard quarterly period. Large businesses account for VAT on a monthly basis. The return will calculate the VAT due as the difference between the total output tax and the deductible input tax. The total value of sales and purchases in the quarter will also have to be entered on the form.

The VAT can be calculated from VAT inclusive figures by multiplying the gross figure by 7/47. For example:

$$\text{Gross daily takings of } £470 \times 7/47 = £70 \text{ VAT}$$

Failure to submit this return on time with the appropriate payment leads to a surcharge liability warning followed by a system of escalating penalty default surcharges. These are capable of crippling a business; it is vital, therefore, to make returns and payment of VAT on time.

Annual accounting scheme

A special scheme is available for small businesses that regularly pay VAT provided that they have been registered for at least a year and the value of their taxable supplies is below £300 000 a year.

An estimate is made from the previous year and nine interim monthly payments will be made by direct debit from your bank. At the end of the year there will be a two-month period to submit the annual return and make any balancing payment.

Special schemes for retailers

There are five special schemes for retailers which apply where a large number of small cash transactions take place and are therefore appropriate in a small animal veterinary practice where both goods and services are supplied to the public.

Point of sale schemes are designed for traders who supply sales and services at both the standard rate and the zero rate. The old retail Scheme F is likely to be the best scheme to adopt but the choice between these schemes will depend on the amount of goods or services you supply at a zero rate of tax. Veterinary practices do occasionally supply zero rated services such as export services for overseas clients.

These retail schemes mean that you do not need to issue separate invoices for each transaction as the VAT can be calculated from the gross takings. The advantages are that there is less record keeping and no payment of VAT is due until the money is actually received – so you are not paying on bad debts.

In a mixed practice it is possible to combine a special scheme with the ordinary accounting method but if more than half your income is derived from non-cash transactions then approval will have to be sought from the local VAT office to adopt a special scheme for the whole of your practice.

Cash accounting scheme

This scheme allows for small businesses with an annual turnover not exceeding £350 000 to account for VAT on the basis of payments received rather than tax invoices.

Like the Retailers Scheme the VAT is not accounted for until the payment has been received. However input tax can only be claimed if the supplier has actually been paid as compared with the standard accounting method which allows you to claim for input tax as soon as the invoice is received – whether it has been paid or not.

Whichever type of scheme you adopt in your practice it is vitally important that you obtain, record and keep all your input invoices including petrol, laundry, cleaning, subsistence meals and even the smaller petty cash items such as pencils and paper clips. You can only claim back the VAT if you can produce a purchase invoice.

Motoring expenses

A taxable person may not deduct VAT, as input tax, on the purchase of motor vehicles unless they are classified as commercial vehicles or vans (a van has no roofed accommodation to the rear of the driver's seat fitted with side windows). Car fuel scale charges are for VAT on fuel used for private motoring in business cars over a three month period. These apply both to employees who have private use of a business car and also to sole proprietors or partners who use fuel for private motoring irrespective of the amount of private motoring undertaken.

Cylinder capacity	Scale charge	VAT due on vehicle
1400 cc or less	£256.00	£38.12
1401 cc to 2000 cc	£325.00	£48.40
More than 2000 cc	£475.00	£71.19

Irrespective of the amount of private motoring undertaken, quarterly scale charges for petrol vehicles apply from 6 April 1996, as shown opposite below.

If you decide to pay the scale charge then you claim back the VAT on the purchase of all your road fuel for both private and business use. If you do only a small amount of private motoring then you need not apply these scale charges but you must buy your own petrol for private motoring and not claim back the VAT on private petrol invoices. Remember that officially travel between a person's home and normal workplace is classed as private motoring.

The VAT inspector

Your local VAT inspector will want to pay you a visit from time to time. They will wish to see that your VAT records have been kept in good order and in particular ask to see all your invoices for which you are claiming back input VAT. It is a good idea to number these invoices and then they can be kept filed in numerical order for ease of reference.

The inspector will ask searching questions to ascertain if all the goods and services shown on these invoices are strictly for business use. In particular he will be looking at the invoices from veterinary wholesale companies for private use items, private use of motoring and telephone, etc. Any discrepancy found may lead the inspector to recover a VAT tax charge and if serious could lead to penalties.

Criminal offences and penalties

Customs and Excise officers may enter and search business premises at any reasonable time for the purpose of exercising their statutory powers. For conviction of the criminal offence of fraudulent evasion of VAT there is an unlimited fine and imprisonment not exceeding seven years. Failure to pay the VAT due, or to furnish a return, can lead to penalties of a default surcharge of 15%, a penalty of £15 a day plus default interest on the sum involved.

Anyone who is dissatisfied with a decision of the Commissioners with respect to the tax has a right of appeal to a VAT tribunal.

Bad debt relief

At the introduction of VAT, bad debt relief could only be claimed on the formal insolvency of the debtor, but these rules were changed by the Finance Act 1990.

The new rules now state that any debt, which is more than six months old, and has been written off in the business accounts, will be eligible for relief from VAT. A write off, which can occur at any time, is defined as the transfer of the debt from the VAT account to a separate bad debt account.

Retail export scheme

The rules pertaining to export are complicated, and only a brief description can be made here. It is suggested that professional advice be sought before embarking on an exporting programme.

Exports of goods and services to another EU country can be made by VAT registered businesses at zero rate, provided that the customer is registered for VAT and that this VAT registration number is shown on the invoice and there is evidence of export.

Exports to overseas countries, other than the EU, can be made at zero rate, provided the goods are exported from the UK within three months, as freight or by post and a valid certificate of export is held.

Summary

Since the introduction of VAT there have been a number of attempts to simplify the paperwork required for the record keeping and the making of the necessary VAT returns. There is however still resentment from small businesses who are acting as unpaid tax collectors for the government.

VAT is here to stay and the closer our ties to the European Union the more likely that this tax will be applied to a wider range of goods, i.e. food, books and children's clothing.

The introduction of VAT did, however, have the benefit that many practices were forced to improve their bookkeeping methods and cash flow with the adoption of improved financial controls within their practices.

Chapter 33
PAYE and National Insurance
John Gripper

All employers of staff are responsible for the deduction of income tax through the Pay As You Earn (PAYE) system and also the deduction of National Insurance contributions for the gross earnings of their employees who are paid under Schedule E.

If the employer fails to deduct the tax then he or she is liable, not the employee. The employer will be liable to penalties as well as a requirement to pay over to the Inland Revenue the tax that he or she should have deducted.

When employing staff for the first time you make an application to the Inland Revenue who will send you a large packet of forms which contains:

- tax payable tables
- free pay tables
- instruction sheets
- payslip booklet and envelopes
- deduction working sheet P11
- *Employer's guide to PAYE*
- statutory sick pay rates and notes
- National Insurance contribution tables
- notes on expense payments and benefits for employees
- various additional forms such as P11D, P24T, P45, P46, etc.

This is a forbidding collection of forms and tables that can be very off-putting to the uninitiated. Do not put it aside to gather dust but take the time to read it through carefully so that you can understand it yourself and follow through the instructions.

Even though you may be delegating a member of your staff to complete the forms and make the necessary deductions it is important that you are able to check their work and sign the annual returns as correct. I am surprised that there are still a number of veterinary practices that hand this work over to their accountants and incur unnecessary expense.

PAYE codes

Each employee is allocated a code number which reflects his non-taxable allowances. For the year 2000/01 the single person's allowance was £4385 so their code number was 438.

The last digit of the allowance is replaced by a letter:

❏ L for a single person
❏ H for a married couple's allowance
❏ P and V are for age allowance, and
❏ K is the code where the employee has taxable benefits of greater value than his personal allowance.

In addition there are letter codes which are used without numbers:

❏ BR means that no allowances have been given and tax should be deducted at basic rate.
❏ NT is the code when no tax is to be deducted.
❏ D (plus number) is for when tax is to be deducted at higher rates.

As well as the personal allowance the employee may claim for other tax reductions which may affect his code number, e.g. personal pensions, maintenance payments, some loan interest and special expenses such as professional subscriptions.

Moving jobs

When an employee moves to a new job he should obtain and bring with him a copy of Parts 2 and 3 of his P45 (details of an employee leaving) which sets out his existing code number and also details of the salary and tax paid for the year to date.

If there is no P45, the new employer must apply for a coding and in the meantime use the emergency code (single person's allowance number) until notification is received from the Inland Revenue on a form P6 which states the code number that should be used for the new employee.

Taxing of benefits

Higher paid employees, who earn more than £8500 a year, are taxed on the benefit of use of car, telephone and accommodation. The employer has to enter the value of the benefits on a Form P11D with his end of year return.

The figure of £8500 also includes the value of the benefits so that an employee earning £8000 a year with a car benefit of, say, £600 a year would have to have a Form P11D completed.

For an employee who is not a higher paid employee, then the benefits, expenses and payments in kind have to be entered on a Form P9D.

Any employee, whatever the level of earnings, who is provided with living accommodation will be liable to tax on an amount equal to the rent, rates and expenses such as heating, lighting, upkeep of garden and domestic help, unless they can claim exemption.

To claim exemption or 'non-beneficial occupation' the Revenue must be satisfied that the accommodation helps the employee to perform their duties better. The Revenue have accepted that in a veterinary practice it is customary to provide accommodation for their employees. It is helpful to have written into the contract of employment of the assistant or nurse that they should live in a certain property as a condition of employment so as to perform his or her duties properly.

Even if employees qualify for exemption they will still be assessed on some of the benefits of the accommodation such as heating, lighting, cleaning and upkeep of the garden, etc., and the use of assets such as television and video (provided that these do not exceed 10% of the net amount of emoluments of the employment).

National Insurance (NI)

There are four main classes of National Insurance contributions:

Class 1: Anyone who works for an employer under a contract of service is liable for payment of Class 1 National Insurance provided they are aged between 16 and 65. This payment is graduated according to the level of earnings above a lower earnings level of £66 per week and below a higher earnings level of £500 a week (2000/01).

If an employee works for more than one employer and the jobs are separate and distinct, then there is liability for NI contributions for each job but no payment need be made in either or both jobs if the earnings do not reach or exceed the lower earnings level.

The 2000/01 rate for the employer is 12.2% on all earnings over the earnings threshold (£84.00 per week for 2000/01) with no maximum.

An employer may contract his employees out of the state scheme benefits if he or she provides a satisfactory occupational scheme. The contracted-out rates are 3% less for salary related schemes (1.6% for money purchase schemes).

Class 1A: NI contributions also have to be paid by employers on the taxable benefit of company cars and car fuel if this car is available for private use by the employee. This payment is based on the value of the car and the level of the business mileage.

Class 2: An individual who is self-employed is liable for payment of a flat rate Class 2 weekly contribution of £6.55 (2000/01) on his earnings provided that they are above the lower earnings limit (£3840 for 1999/00).

This is normally paid by direct debit through a bank. Application may be made for deferment of Class 2 contributions until such time as it is possible to calculate the exact liability.

An employer need make no deductions for National Insurance or PAYE for a worker who is self-employed, i.e. locums or short-term assistants. However the employer must be satisfied that the local tax office has accepted that the locum is self-employed and written evidence should be produced by the locum to confirm his status.

Instances have occurred where veterinary surgeons have accepted assurances from the locum as to his self-employed status and paid him gross fees – only to find that when an inspector from the DSS has made a visit, that it had not had official sanction. It is then the employer that is liable to pay back all the NI and income tax that should have been deducted – and they may go back six years.

Class 3: This is a voluntary contribution paid at a flat rate which may be paid in order to qualify for NI benefits, e.g. persons who have been working abroad.

Class 4: This is an earnings related contribution for self-employed persons only and is paid on the profits of the business. In 2000/01 the rate was 6% and was paid on profits between £4385 and £27 820. This tax is assessed and collected by the Inland Revenue along with Schedule D income tax.

Deduction working sheet

The deduction working sheet (P11) should be completed every week or month by the employer for each employee who is paid more than the minimum earnings rate for National Insurance. An immediate saving in secretarial time can be achieved by insisting that all your employees are paid monthly and by cheque.

All the payments for the month for both National Insurance and PAYE are entered into the payslip booklet (P30BC). These are added up and sent with a cheque to the Collector of Taxes on a monthly or quarterly basis.

You can computerise your payroll with a software package which will take away much of the hard work. Such a program will produce for you each month a comprehensive wage slip and show all the deductions.

End of year returns

After 5 April you have to send in your end of year returns. Each employee has to be given a copy of a P14 which shows the total tax and National Insurance that has been deducted from his earnings during the year. The employer adds up the totals of the P14 forms and enters them on the annual statement (P35), and returns it along with a cheque with any under payment which may have been made during the year.

If you have any casual employees or part-time employees who have not needed a P14 then you must include them on a Form P38. Your annual return will also include the benefits and expenses forms P9D and the dreaded P11D.

Chapter 34

Insurance and Pensions

John Gripper

Insurance offers protection against a possible loss. Assurance provides for the payment of a sum of money in the future, for example on the maturity of an endowment policy.

The richer you are the less you need take out insurance – there seems little point in insuring your camera against loss when you can afford to buy a replacement. As an individual you have to take out a house protection policy against the loss of your home from fire; yet a large property company or local authority that owned hundreds of houses might decide to accept its own insurance risks rather than pay premiums to an insurance company.

The decision as to which types of insurance, assurance and pension policies you need to take out should be a matter of discussion with your insurance broker, combined with a common sense approach to meet your own particular financial and personal circumstances.

Professional negligence insurance

Professional negligence insurance has now been made compulsory by the RCVS for any veterinary surgeon who is in practice. As a veterinary assistant it will be the responsibility of your employer to take out professional negligence insurance to cover any claims made against you – so check that your practice has adequate cover. As soon as you are self-employed it then becomes your own responsibility to take out cover against claims of professional negligence.

Premiums for the veterinary profession are still relatively modest but if the number and size of claims continue to rise as the public becomes more litigious, then we can expect increases in premiums in line with other professionals, i.e. accountants, lawyers and doctors.

A small number of commercial companies offer this type of negligence insurance but the majority of veterinary surgeons obtain their professional indemnity cover through membership of the Veterinary Defence Society, an insurance company formed and managed by members of the veterinary profession.

There is a sliding scale of premiums to match the levels and types of cover required. If you decide to take out cover elsewhere read the small print very carefully to ensure that you and all your staff (including locums and students) are fully protected, that the policy includes the full legal costs of defending a claim, and that there is not an aggregation limit on the number of claims that can be made.

The growing concern within the professions over ever-increasing claims from the public and the need to practise defensive medicine have led to demands for the introduction of limited liability status for practices accompanied by mandatory professional negligence insurance.

A new insurance policy called the Veterinary Legal Expenses Insurance Scheme has now been launched whereby the veterinary surgeon can obtain cover for legal costs for prosecutions in criminal courts resulting from normal professional work or for an appearance before the RCVS Disciplinary Committee.

Costs incurred in respect of a summons to appear before the RCVS Disciplinary Committee and for a barrister or solicitor to be present at the hearing to present his defence will be payable whatever the outcome of the hearing, subject to a maximum of £50 000. For a criminal prosecution resulting from normal professional work, the insurance will pay the costs only if the defendant is eventually found not guilty.

Health insurance

Permanent health insurance

As a young professional, with a lifetime career ahead of you, it is important that you take out protection against the event of long-term sickness or disability which can prevent you earning a living from your chosen profession. This can be done by means of a permanent health or continuous disability insurance policy that is non-cancellable and will pay you an income for the rest of your working life should you suffer long-term ill-health.

The level of premiums relates to the length of the benefit deferred period – the premiums for payment for being off ill after a week will be considerably higher than one stipulating a waiting period of a month or three months. Assistants' contracts of employment will stipulate the period that salaries will continue to be paid by the practice for illness and accident so that cover can be taken for an appropriate waiting period.

Those practitioners who have entered into a partnership will find that the partnership contract will usually provide for some protection for short-term illness or disability but that after an agreed period the individual partner becomes responsible for the payment of a locum. Eventually a termination of the partnership will take place if the absence from work is prolonged. A permanent health policy with an appropriate benefit waiting period can be taken out by each partner to protect a part of their income.

Benefits will continue to be paid until you return to work or reach retirement age. It is important to ensure that the policy pays up if you cannot work within your own profession and does not insist that you have to earn a living in alternative work such as a car park attendant.

Critical illness

A critical illness policy pays out a lump sum if the insured is diagnosed as suffering from a potentially terminal condition or total disability. There are problems over the insurer's standard definitions of what constitutes a critical illness and care should be taken to read the small print and select the right policy.

It is possible with a critical illness policy to collect the lump sum, to have the corrective treatment or surgery, recover, and then return to work.

Medical insurance

There are a large variety of medical policies available which may cover full hospital treatment and consultants' fees or just compensation for days spent in hospital (which nowadays may be quite short).

Medical insurance is regarded by some as a luxury or just queue jumping the National Health Service waiting lists, but for the self-employed it is very important that you receive the appropriate medical and surgical treatment at a time and place that is convenient to yourself and your practice without delay.

Life insurance

You may need life insurance cover under certain circumstances – the cheapest form is term insurance which provides cover for a stated period and therefore the premium is lower than full life insurance that pays out on your death.

Since the advent of AIDS, life insurance premiums have risen and some companies have withdrawn convertible term assurance; however many companies have now excluded payment for death from AIDS related conditions.

If you take out a loan or a mortgage then the bank or building society will ask you to also take out an insurance policy against your early death so as to protect their investment. This could be term insurance or whole life (which will continue until terminated by your death).

You may choose to take out an endowment policy which will be either 'with profits' or a 'non profit' policy and will pay out a lump sum at a pre-determined maturity date or on your earlier death. The 'with profits' endowment insurance can also provide a useful investment as compared with the 'non-profit' which will only return the pre-arranged sum at maturity.

It is commonplace within a partnership agreement to state that each of the partners shall take out a cross insurance policy under trust to cover the life of each partner so that in the event of the death of a partner then the remaining partners will receive a capital sum available to pay out to the spouse or the estate of the deceased partner.

When you have the responsibility of a young family it is prudent to provide an income for them in the event of your death. This can be arranged by means of a family income policy that will provide your spouse and children with a continuing income after your death.

Practice surgery policy

A comprehensive practice policy will cover your surgery premises, veterinary instruments and equipment, business machines (including computers) and stocks of drugs against fire, theft and other risks. Cover through an all risks policy can also include loss of profits in the event of a major disruption to your business.

The Employers' Liability (Compulsory Insurance) Act 1969 prescribes that all employers must insure against liability for personal injury or disease sustained by their employees arising out of, or in the course of, their employment in Great Britain.

The amount of insurance cover that must be taken out is cover for at least £10 million in respect of any claim, arising out of one occurrence. For every day that the employer is not insured he may be liable for summary conviction and a fine up to £2500. A copy of the insurance certificate must be displayed at each place of business or the employer may be liable to a fine of £1000.

Most practice comprehensive policies will include employers' liability insurance cover against claims from members of the public for personal injuries and also liability for animals in care or custody including accidental escape of animals (but not indemnity against professional negligence).

Motor insurance

Motor insurance is compulsory against claims for third party, fire and theft risks and this is often all that is required for cars of low value. However, most veterinary surgeons will take out fully comprehensive insurance policies for their motor cars.

There are a great variety of companies offering this type of motor insurance at different rates, so shop around for quotations, including the direct line offers. Remember that the best motor insurance company is not always the one with the cheapest premiums but is the one that will pay out at the time of a claim without undue hassle or delay.

Generous 'no claim' discounts up to 70% can be built up but it usually takes three years of accident free driving to reach the maximum. A more recent additional option that has been available is the 'protected no claim discount' which for a small increase in premium allows you to make a claim but still protects your no claim discount in the event of an accident.

Particular problems arise for young people under 26 years of age who find that their premiums are heavily loaded – especially if they want to drive soft top sports cars.

A continuing source of annoyance is the loss of your no claims bonus discount for a claim where the accident was not your fault but the insurance company has operated the 'knock for knock' intercompany agreement.

In addition to your normal motor insurance you can take out with the AA or RAC or Green Flag a rescue and recovery policy that will ensure that you do not get stranded if your car breaks down, which can be expensive if it happens on a motorway.

State retirement pensions

The basic weekly 'old age' state retirement pension for 2000/01 is £107.90 for a married couple and £67.50 for a single person. This pension can be taken at the age of 65 for men and 60 for single women. Married women have to wait until their husband reaches age 65, unless they are entitled to a state pension in their own right. This pension is usually adjusted upwards each year at Budget time to keep in line with inflation. There is an option to postpone the pension should you wish to continue working after retirement age. The pension will then increase by increments of 7.5% each year until the age of 70 for men.

An additional pension from the government is SERPS (State Earnings Related Pension Scheme). Contributions will have been paid to SERPS out of National Insurance deductions by all employees who are not in a 'contracted out' company scheme. The government now wish to reduce their commitment under the SERPS scheme. After the year 2000 the benefits will be reduced and new pension legislation encourages more employees to make their own private pension arrangements.

The attractions of contracting out of SERPS vary according to your age. This is because the level of rebate is the same whatever the age, but the cost of buying the benefit increases with age. That means that people near to retirement will almost certainly be better off remaining in SERPS, whereas younger employees under, say age 45, might possibly be expected to benefit by contracting out of SERPS into a private pension plan. Once again, professional advice should always be sought.

If an employee takes out an appropriate private pension plan, both employer and employee pay the normal rate of National Insurance contributions. The DSS will then pay direct to the pension plan a sum equal to the contracting out rebate, which varies according to the type of scheme, together with income tax due on the employee's share.

Personal pensions

Personal pension schemes have been available for the self-employed for many years but have now been extended to the employed as well. Such schemes will provide at the time of retirement a tax free lump sum with an absolute maximum of £150 000 per policy and also a pension annuity.

The premiums for these policies are invested in a tax free fund and there are three types of plan available:

(1) *Unit Linked*: Premiums are invested directly into your choice of unit trust. The invested fund will rise or fall depending on the success or failure of your chosen unit trust, in line with the stock market performance, after allowing for the expenses and commission of the insurance company.

(2) *With Profits*: The premiums are invested in a broader range of investments by the insurance company. On retirement the pension is made up of a guaranteed pension plus a revisionary bonus and sometimes also a terminal bonus which is related to the overall performance of the insurance company.

(3) *Deposit Scheme*: The amount of the fund at the time is the total of the premiums paid into the fund plus a fixed rate of interest which may be variable but is in line with the deposit interest rate. A deposit scheme is more suitable for someone who has only a short period to retirement and does not wish to be associated with the risk of stock market fluctuations.

If you are aged 35 or younger 17.5% of net relevant earnings can be paid into a personal pension plan. Above that age there is a sliding scale which allows a higher percentage of contributions, and at age 61 or over you can contribute 40% of your net relevant earnings.

The benefits can be taken from the age of 50 without actually having to retire. When you choose to take your pension annuity there is an open market option which allows you to shop around and select the best annuity available on the market from your pension fund. You will also have to decide the type of annuity which you require. There are now many choices which will be influenced by current annuity rates, your age and available income.

❒ Do you want a joint annuity that provides for a two thirds pension for your spouse on your death?
❒ Do you want a fixed rate annuity or an escalating annuity at the rate of 3% or 5%, or even an annuity that is linked to RPI (retail price index)?
❒ Do you want one that is investment linked (this could be 'with profits' or directly linked to a unit trust)?

New flexible annuities have now been introduced for personal pensions which allow the pensioners to withdraw some income from their existing fund before cashing in the annuity. If you have a number of different policies you can design your own phasing programme and cash in segments or different policies over a period but up to a maximum age of 75 years. Professional advice can be obtained from an insurance broker on these annuity decisions.

It is now possible to use your pension for 'loan back' schemes which allow you to borrow money for house purchase or business loans such as practice purchase. This is a very efficient method of borrowing: you pay the pension premiums and the interest on the loan but the capital sum of money is paid back on the maturity of the policy when the tax free sum becomes available.

Company pension schemes

These are either 'final salary' or 'money purchase' schemes. The final salary scheme will guarantee you a fixed pension related to each year of service and is linked to your final salary whilst the money purchase scheme pension is dependent on the performance of the fund into which your premiums have been invested.

As a member of a company pension scheme you have a choice of staying with the company scheme or changing to an appropriate personal pension scheme. Do not leave your company pension scheme until you have carefully weighed up the full implications and taken independent financial advice.

It is possible to stay within the company pension scheme and pay free-standing additional voluntary contributions (FSAVCs) to a private pension scheme with premiums of up to 15% of your earnings.

The government proposes to introduce a new 'stakeholder' pension in 2001. This has been designed as a cheaper and simpler type of pension available where there are five or more employees. The employer must offer employees this scheme, but need not make any contribution to the premiums.

Financial Services Act

The Financial Services Act came into force in April 1988. It is an offence for anyone who is not registered under the Act to give specific advice on insurance or investments. In order to register it is necessary to be licensed by the Personal Investment Authority.

Before the financial adviser can advise you he must know his customer, provide 'best advice', be competent and undertake research and survey the market. The financial adviser must retain records to show that he or she has abided by these regulations.

Under the polarisation requirements of the Act there are two main types of advisers or intermediaries selling life insurance and investments:

(1)   *Tied advisers* who are only able to advise and sell the products of one company. This type of advice is found in the clearing banks, building societies and insurance companies.

(2) *Independent advisers* who act as insurance brokers and are free to advise and select the products of any insurance company.

It is now obligatory for all financial advisers to declare to their client the commission that they will receive from a policy sale.

Chapter 35

Pharmacy

Peter Gripper

Pharmacy covers a wide range of topics including the fabric of the building, stock itself, storage conditions, stock management, record keeping, auditing, dispensing and labelling. Stock control and management are covered elsewhere in this book but it is worth repeating that good stock management is an integral part of good pharmacy and this includes stock ordering, stock levels, storage, stock rotation, dispensing and disposal. Each practice should have a proper stock rotation policy so that all stock is used in the correct order (first in – first out).

There must be a named person in each practice who is responsible for medicines and pharmacy and this named person must ensure that the medicines legislation is observed correctly and that the requisite records are kept correctly. They also are responsible for the procedures and protocols related to dispensing and pharmacy within the practice.

The Medicines Act 1968 provides that veterinarians can retail prescription only medicines (POM), pharmacy and merchants' list (PML) and pharmacy (P) products provided that they are administered by them or under their direction to animals under their care. The Medicines Act 1968 also gives veterinary surgeons the privilege to dispense, but the right to prescribe is conferred due to membership of the Royal College of Veterinary Surgeons (RCVS).

The premises used for the pharmacy should be a solid permanent structure which is secure against vermin and vandals. Ideally it should be lockable and access to the pharmacy restricted to those persons trained in dispensing and pharmacy. The room should allow for appropriate temperature control to store the various products and some form of monitoring to ensure that temperatures remain within the defined boundaries.

All incoming stock should be checked on arrival and the batch number and expiry date recorded. Any short dated stock should not be accepted. The expiry dates of stock on the shelf should also be checked regularly, e.g. monthly, and any out of date stock disposed of as pharmaceutical waste.

Dispensing

Local rules should be written for dispensing and all staff who are responsible for dispensing should be trained in the tasks they will be expected to undertake. This will cover the legal as well as the practical aspects of dispensing. The labelling requirements and practice protocols for dispensing and record keeping must be followed and staff should have been trained in the handling of medicines.

Dispensing staff should be familiar with the different legal categories of medicines, (POM, P, PML and general sales list (GSL)) and know which product groups can be dispensed, under what circumstances and to whom. POM, P and PML products can only be dispensed upon the authority of a veterinary surgeon and only to a bona fide client for animals under the veterinary surgeon's care.

The definition of 'animals under their care' in the *RCVS Guide to Professional Conduct* is as follows.

❑ The veterinarian should have been given responsibility for the health of the animal or herd in question by the owner or the owner's agent.
❑ The care of the animal or herd by the veterinarian should be real not merely nominal.
❑ The veterinarian should at least
  ■ either have seen the animal or herd for the purpose of diagnosis and prescription and immediately prior thereto or
  ■ have visited the farm or other premises in which the animal or herd is kept sufficiently often and recently enough to have acquired from personal knowledge and inspection an accurate and up to date picture of the health status of that farm sufficient to enable him or her to make a diagnosis and prescribe for the animal or herd in question.

Categories of medicines have different requirements for supply. Prescription only medicines can only be supplied by or against written authority of a veterinary prescription. Pharmacy can be supplied by a registered pharmacist over the counter or by a veterinary surgeon for animals under their care.

Pharmacy and merchants' list medicines can be supplied

❑ by a pharmacist to any customer
❑ by an agricultural merchant (registered with the Royal Pharmaceutical Society of Great Britain (RPSGB) to any keeper of animals but only for the correct species under the licence
❑ by a veterinary surgeon for animals under their care *only* to their own clients
❑ by a registered saddler to persons who have horses or ponies in their charge
❑ a sub division of the PML list allows certain dealers to sell by retail a small range of equine products to the public.

General sales list medicines can be sold without any restriction over the counter and the saddlers' list permits registered saddlers to sell the limited range of horse wormers.

Labelling

Any product dispensed should be labelled correctly and clearly. Either the container or the outer package must be labelled and labels should carry any specific warnings for the client. The labels should be completed in biro, roller ball or felt tip but ink and pencil are not allowed. If possible, mechanical labelling is preferable and computer systems that generate labels do allow automatic inclusion of warnings and withdrawal periods on the labels.

If the product insert leaflet is intended for the final user then it should be left with the container. The information that should appear on the label includes:

- name of owner
- name and address of veterinary surgeon
- date
- name of medicine
- strength of medicine
- batch number
- dose to be given and directions for use
- name of animal to be treated
- the wording 'For animal treatment only'*
- the wording 'Keep out of reach of children'*
- the wording 'For external use only'* if applicable
- relevant withdrawal periods for food producing animals
- relevant warnings for operator.

* These do not have to appear on the veterinary surgeon's label if they already appear on the container supplied by the manufacturer.

EU legislation requires the following details to be kept for each incoming and outgoing transaction of medicine:

- date
- product
- batch number
- quantity received and supplier
- quantity supplied and to whom
- name of recipient
- prescribing veterinary surgeon's details.

The practice should conduct a full audit, at least annually, on supply and usage of pharmaceutical products.

Containers

When medicines are prepared from bulk then they should be packaged as follows:

- coloured fluted bottles – for all external applications
- plain glass bottles – for cough mixtures or tonics
- wide mouthed jars – for creams, powders and ointments
- opaque containers – for light sensitive medicines
- child-resistant containers – for all solid oral formulations.

Tablets should be put into containers that protect against crushing, breakage, moisture, contamination and deterioration. Paper envelopes are not suitable as the sole packing except for blister packs and foil wrapped tablets. Discretion is allowed when dispensing to people who may have difficulty opening child-resistant containers, for example people with arthritis.

Controlled drugs

These have their own set of rules regarding supply and record keeping under the following legislation.

- Misuse of Drugs Act 1971
- Misuse of Drugs Regulations 1985
- Medicines Act 1968.

Controlled drugs (CD) are divided into five categories. Schedule I includes cannabis and hallucinogenics e.g. LSD. These are supplied only under special licence and have no therapeutic veterinary uses. I shall not discuss these further.

Schedule 2 includes cocaine, heroin, Immobilon, fentanyl and pethidine. They are only available on special prescription and requisition requirements have to be met. They have to be kept in an approved CD cabinet and in safe custody and full records must be kept by the veterinary surgeon, of arrivals and use, in a bound CD register. Any destruction of unwanted or out of date product has to be authorised and also to be witnessed by a representative of the Home Office. Records of destruction of product should be entered in the CD register. Schedule 2 drugs must be kept in a locked cabinet, the key to which is only held by veterinary surgeons. The practice should only stock the minimum required in the practice.

Schedule 3 includes barbiturates, buprenorphine and a few stimulants. These are subject to less stringent controls but do need prescriptions and requisition orders. However, transactions do not have to be recorded in the register. Some have to be kept in a locked cabinet. There are no special destruction requirements.

Schedule 4 includes Valium, Librium, and benzodiazepines. There are no special requirements for these products for veterinary surgeons.

Schedule 5 includes codeine and pholcodine. The rules for these products mainly relate to manufacture of the preparations for industry.

Supply of controlled drugs
Schedule 2 and 3 can be obtained from your wholesaler or manufacturer or pharmacist on a requisition order which details your name and address and profession. The veterinary surgeon must sign it, state the purpose they are required for and the total quantity required.

Storage of controlled drugs
Schedule 2 drugs need to be in a locked cabinet, Schedule 3 and 4 do not. The keys should be held by veterinary surgeons only. Motor cars are not considered a locked receptacle unless there is a CD cabinet bolted to the chassis of the vehicle. Stocks should not be kept in practice vehicles and on visits great care must be taken of any supplies carried.

Records for controlled drugs
The rules for recording the storage and prescription of controlled drugs are stringent.

- Records must be completed within 24 hours in a bound book used solely for CDs.
- Each premises that stores CDs must have its own book and a separate part of the book should be used for each product.
- Entries must be made in chronological order and be indelible.
- Any alterations should be made in the margins or underneath; no writing should be obscured and no correction fluids used.
- Records must be kept for two years from the date of the last entry.
- Date of supply or receipt should be noted including
  - name and address of the owner
  - quantity
  - strength
  - product
  - reason for use.

As with all products there is not only a legal responsibility for the veterinary surgeon but also a moral responsibility. There are certain products subject to abuse or potential misuse that would benefit from safer storage but which do not appear on the above schedules.

Cascade

The Medicines Regulations define the protocol to be used when prescribing and state that

'no person shall administer or cause or permit to be administered any veterinary medicinal product to an animal unless a product licence has been granted under the act in respect of that product'

When prescribing, the following options should be considered in order, to assist in the selection of appropriate medication.

❐ Option 1: a product that is licensed for that species and that condition
❐ Option 2: a product that is licensed for another condition in the same species
❐ Option 3: a product that is licensed for use in another species can be prescribed
❐ Option 4: a product that is licensed for human administration
❐ Option 5: special product made up under veterinary prescription by an authorised person.

In food producing animals, Options 3, 4 or 5 only apply when treating a small number of animals. The Veterinary Medicine Directorate (VMD) have issued guidance as to what they consider is a 'small number' of animals.

For Options 2, 3, 4 and 5 products may contain only substances to be found in licensed products for food animal species. They must be administered by a vet or under their direction, and adequate records kept by the vet (see above).

If the cascade is not followed, then the veterinary surgeon must have written records regarding the decision process and keep these notes for three years, recording

❐ date of examination
❐ name and address of owner
❐ number of animals treated
❐ diagnosis
❐ product prescribed
❐ dose administered
❐ duration of treatment
❐ recommended withdrawal period.

A consent form can also be used for owners to sign when products are used outside the data sheet, as will be the case when treating exotic pets and most small rodents and rabbits (note that rabbits can also be food producing animals). In the event that a product is used without the data sheet recommendation then standard withdrawal periods apply unless the veterinary surgeon has data to the contrary. The standard withdrawal periods are

❐ 7 days for eggs
❐ 7 days for milk
❐ 28 days for meat
❐ 500° (Celcius) days for meat from fish.

Where a product is used 'off licence' a record should be kept for three years as to why that product was used as well as the usual details.

The *RCVS Guide to Professional Conduct*, Chapter 3 and the *BVA Code of Practice on Medicines* are good references and offer further guidance with regard to regulations on pharmacy.

Chapter 36

Health and Safety and COSHH (Control of Substances Hazardous to Health)

Peter Gripper

COSHH is a very broad subject which encompasses many regulations. This chapter outlines the principles of the COSHH regulations and how they apply to veterinary practices and it also covers health and safety issues and risk assessments.

The Control of Substances Hazardous to Health (COSHH) Regulations define hazardous materials as follows.

(1) Any product with an occupational exposure standard. The Health and Safety Executive (HSE) publish a booklet (EH40) with the complete list of products and this is updated annually. Chemicals such as formaldehyde and pharmaceuticals such as halothane and isoflurane are included in this list.
(2) Hazardous microorganisms.
(3) Dust at a level that could promote or initiate asthma.
(4) Other hazardous chemicals. This includes not only pharmaceutical products but also laboratory chemicals and cleaning materials. This latter area is often overlooked in practices.

Where a risk exists, the legislation places an employer under a duty to identify the risk and lessen it if possible. This may mean the use of an alternative product of lower risk. Protective clothing must be provided if necessary. Under the regulations every employer should do the following.

❐ *Produce a COSHH assessment:* this should be a written assessment for the practice.
❐ *Reduce any risks, where possible:* this involves risk assessment to establish the level of risk and identify ways of reducing those risks.
❐ *Make employees aware of the risks and the assessment:* the assessments must be available for members of the practice so should be stored somewhere where there is easy access for everyone in the practice. New staff should be provided with copies of the assessments on joining the practice and these should be explained as part of their induction programme.
❐ *Monitor the assessment and update it:* a system should be in place to ensure that regular monitoring and reviews occur. The COSHH and health and safety assessments should be reviewed at least annually. There should also be a review if there are new products or procedures introduced into the practice.

The main emphasis is on reducing exposure to a risk, or removing it completely by substituting a safer alternative product. The use of protective clothing is the last resort and not the first action you take.

An individual within the practice must be appointed COSHH officer and it is their role to coordinate the assessment and any future updating and monitoring. One of the major parts of the legal obligation is that once produced the COSHH assessment has to be updated and monitored regularly.

Once you have produced the assessment then it is imperative that you implement it and ensure that everyone in the practice knows not only of its existence but also of its content. Memos circulated to all staff with a copy on the safety notice board ensure everyone knows about any new rules, procedures or hazards. It is also a good idea to obtain signatures from staff that they have read and understood the assessment. This gives an opportunity to discuss any contentious areas and ensures that everyone is of the same opinion whilst also emphasising the importance that you attach to the assessment.

Devising a COSHH assessment

As part of your COSHH assessment, all medicines and drugs should be assessed by some method and then classified. There is no single method which is better than any other but my own practice has tried to produce a system that is simple and easy to understand. This means that it is also easy and quick to update and all staff within the premises can understand the implications of the classification. It begins by listing the drugs and chemicals into three main appendices.

(1)   Those producets classified under the CHIP (Chemical Hazardous Information and Packaging) Regulations. These oblige us to address safety of chemicals that we supply, including ones we make up within the premises. For home-made remedies and other similar recipes handed down over the years, it is up to us, as formulators, to assess the safety of the final product from its known constituents and to label it accordingly.

(2)   This second group is classified by pharmaceutical action and includes products that are potentially harmful. It includes categories such as
     ❐   cardiac preparations
     ❐   sedatives
     ❐   stimulants
     ❐   anaesthetics
     ❐   narcotics
     ❐   hormones
     ❐   vaccines, particularly oil based products
     ❐   perceutaneously absorbed products
     ❐   cytotoxic and teratogenic products.

(3)   The third category of products is those that are 'harmless in normal use . . .' but does of course accept that any product can be harmful to any individual that shows hypersensitivity to that particular product.

Fortunately there is plenty of information available to help you assess the drugs. The safety data sheet (SDS) provided, on request, by the manufacturing company is the starting point and these are detailed and specific. They follow a standard format and have details on handling and saftey measures and they also include advice on first aid and spillage procedures. The product data sheet in the NOAH compendium also may have some information and directions on safety, but it is not as comprehensive as the safety data sheet. The manufacturing company concerned can also be contacted direct for further advice.

Once you have assessed products you may have to go a step further with certain products that are hazardous. For those particular products that are potentially harmful local rules have to be written and displayed. These can then be followed by everyone within the practice to ensure the safe use of the product.

The local rules can often be drawn up utilising the information you have collected and should be written with the routine practice procedures in mind. They should be displayed and all staff be aware of them. The rules need not be complicated and should be simple and easy to understand.

Any hazardous products that are dispensed must obviously be dispensed with a warning given to the client and, where necessary, a written copy on how to handle them. Computerised labelling enables many practices to indentify these products and written warnings will automatically appear on the label. For those practices where this does not apply to every single product, you must devise and implement an identification system.

Clinical waste

Clinical waste is defined as:

> 'Any waste which consists wholly or partly of animal tissue, blood or other body fluids, excretions, drugs, pharmaceutical products, swabs or dressings, syringes, needles or other sharp instruments, or any other waste arising from veterinary practice, investigation, treatment, care, teaching or research.'

It is therefore apparent that all medicines, chemicals and clinical waste are included in the COSHH regulations.

All clinical waste must be classified and disposed of according to the current requirement which presently is by incineration. This includes carcases, sharps, clinical waste and also pharmaceutical waste which is a separate category within clinical waste and is defined as 'special waste' with its own set of rules. Firms collecting and disposing of clinical waste must hold licences for transport, disposal and for their site. All waste collected must be accompanied by a consignment note which must be kept for two years. Waste must be securely sealed, identified and kept in cool storage awaiting collection.

It goes without saying that all practices must have suitable protective equipment available for staff to use, such as disposable gloves, plastic aprons, safety spectacles, disposable face masks, an eyewash and first aid kits. Heavy duty gloves, animal catchers and stretchers are also needed.

Other areas of risk

Certain areas and topics need special attention such as ionising radiation which has its own set of regulations. Regulations exist for other areas as well, such as manual handling, first aid and personal protective equipment.

Most practices are familar with the legal requirements of the Ionising Radiation Regulations and ionising radiation is certainly an identified hazard for employees. If all the requirements of the Ionising Radiation Regulations are being implemented and observed then this will also cover nearly all the COSHH and health and safety aspects as well. The practice will have its own guidelines and local rules, will be registered with the local health and safety executive as a user of ionising radiation and will have appointed a Radiation Protection Supervisor (RPS) and a Radiation Protection Advisor (RPA). Personal dosemeters, protective lead aprons, gloves, gowns and warning signs and lights are familar to most veterinary surgeons. Adequate ventilation of automatic processors and full record keeping are also necessary.

As well as ionising radiation, special attention must be given to other areas such as anaesthesia and clinical and pharmaceutical waste. Health and safety policy will cover other areas including refreshments, fire safety, first aid, accident and Reporting of Injury, Diseases and Dangerous Occurrences Regulations (RIDDOR) procedures, autoclaves and other equipment.

A written spillage procedure should be drawn up for cleaning up any spillage and great care should be taken not to injure yourself on any cut glass. Absorbent paper towels or sand are the most suitable materials and these should then be disposed of accordingly. Anaesthesia merits special attention and anasesthetic machines should be serviced to ensure satisfactory and safe functioning.

Scavenging of waste anaesthetic gases must be efficient and effective. Active scavenging is advisable and several tailor made systems now exist for veterinary surgeons. Passive systems are not illegal as long as they work effectively and to this end monitoring of waste gases should be carried out to assess the efficacy of the system. This is another example of ongoing monitoring. Attention should also be given to the recovery room where high levels of volatile anaesthetic agent can collect during the recovery phase.

Health and safety considerations

All veterinary practices need to address their obligations under the current legislation with regard to the management of health and safety at work. Health and safety covers a wide range of topics and the relevant legislation is frequently changed and amended.

The basic principles are similar throughout and the objective is to make the workplace safer, to reduce accidents, and to reduce the risk to employees and visitors to your premises.

The method approved by the Health and Safety Executive (HSE) to address health and safety issues is to use risk assessment and every practice should be familiar with the process of risk assessment and have completed risk assessments. This includes all staff and not just the principal and partners.

For a business or practice that wishes to start from scratch, the first step is to identify the potential hazards in the practice. This can be done by asking each member of staff to identify the three or four main risks in their own particular job, and the three or four main risks in the practice as a whole. The results from all the staff submissions can be collated and the list prioritised. The risks can then be addressed starting with the most important.

All staff should be familiar with and be involved in producing risk assessments. I consider it very important that the individual carrying out a particular task is involved in the assessment of that task because they are the person most familiar with any problems associated with that specific task. The practice owner has overall responsibility but the practice manager or managing partner will oversee the production of risk assessments and put into place systems to monitor and review risk assessments in the workplace.

The risk assessments can be completed in two phases, an initial assessment by the person who carries out the task and their findings then being the basis for discussion and completion of the final assessment.

The risk assessment form can be used to assess a broad range of potential hazards. For example the hazard may be

❐ a *procedure* such as anaesthesia
❐ a *product* such as isoflurane
❐ a *product group* such as oil-adjuvant vaccines
❐ a *task* such as handling fractious animals
❐ *manual handling*
❐ *computer usage and visual display units* (VDU).

A simple form can be produced for the initial assessment and answers be sought to the questions below.

❐ What is the hazard?
❐ Who is at risk?

- How serious is the risk?
- What is the probability of it occurring?
- Is there a risk to staff, visitors or the environment?
- What is the likely outcome of any injury? Major or minor? Fatal?
- Is there any protective equipment needed?
- Is there any special procedure needed for first aid, fire or spillage?
- What control measures are in place?
- Are they effective?
- If current controls are not satisfactory what is needed?
- When will this be done by?
- Who will do it?
- Who monitors this particular risk?
- When should it be reviewed?

I suggest that the practice staff are divided into groups of two or three people and in each group there should be a cross section of staff. A group that consists of a veterinary surgeon, a nurse and a receptionist allows for a variety of views and opinions. Each group has several risk assessments to complete and these can be reviewed by one of the other groups. All risk assessments can then be discussed at staff meetings prior to filing them safely.

The final stage is to monitor and review the risk assessments. They should be reviewed annually at least, and more often if there is a change in the procedure or the products used.

As part of the induction programme for new staff, risk assessments should be discussed and explained and copies provided where necessary. Risk assessments should be kept in one file to which staff have easy access.

There is a lot of legislation that covers health and safety issues and I have listed below a few areas and topics which everyone should address. This is not intended to be an exhaustive checklist but more of a start point. It is not in any priority order.

- visual display units (VDU)
- Electricity at Work Regulations
- manual handling tasks
- first aid
- protective clothing
- Reporting of Injury, Diseases and Dangerous Occurrences Regulations
- pregnancy
- spillage
- anaesthesia
- ionising radiation
- staff contracts
- health and safety policy document.

The risk assessment will help identify areas where improvements could be made and also set a date for completing and implementing those changes.

A Health and Safety Policy Statement should be written and on display for all staff to read. This notice board can then serve as the safety notice board and any new procedures or memos on changes in safety rules can be posted onto this board for all staff to read.

Refreshments must be kept entirely separate from all clinical areas and no tea or coffee is permitted in animal, medicine or laboratory areas. The sinks used for making refreshment and cleaning cups should be entirely separate from any sinks used for washing instruments, clinical work or cleaning animals prior to or after treatments.

All practices should have a fire drill and practise it. Extinguishers should be serviced annually and the local fire officer will advise on the site, type and number of fire extinguishers required. All staff should be aware of the different types of extinguisher and on which fires they can be used.

First aid kits should be of an approved type only and available at the reception desk for use by a client in the event of an accident. They should contain only the dedicated human dressings and the size of the kit should be appropriate to the number of employees. Every practice should have an eyewash for use in emergencies.

The accident book must be kept up to date and all accidents recorded. If the accident is serious or meets one of the listed criteria then it has to be reported under RIDDOR.

The BVA COSHH booklet acts as a reference text on many subjects and should be kept with the COSHH assessment. It details the Maximum Exposure Limits (MEL) and Time Weighted Average (TWA) for certain products.

All equipment must be serviced appropriately and a record kept of when it was done. Any repairs must be completed promptly. For certain equipment the servicing may be as frequently as every six months but most of the equipment needs annual servicing. The manufacturer's instructions on how to operate equipment should be followed for each item and be displayed near the item concerned.

Pregnancy merits special consideration and in the event of a member of staff becoming pregnant then they must inform the COSHH officer and a risk assessment should be carried out. The risk to the unborn child has to be considered and different precautions may be necessary.

Chapter 37

Employment Law

John Gripper

There is a massive framework of legislation that encompasses Employment Law and Individual Rights. The Employment Protection (Consolidation) Act 1978 has 160 sections and 14 Schedules.

Written particulars of terms of employment

As soon as a job has been offered and accepted, a contract of employment comes into effect automatically; the terms may be simply those stated at the interview, or they may be set out by a letter offering or confirming the job.

All new employees (including part-timers) whose employment continues for a month or more must receive a written statement of particulars of employment. This statement must be provided by the employer within two months of the start of work.

There is an important difference between a written contract and a written statement. A contract, whether oral or in writing, is legally binding whereas the written statement of particulars is a statement for information only and sets out the more important terms of the employment.

Every principal statement or contract should provide the following:

❐ names of the employer and employee
❐ date when employment began
❐ scale or rate of pay
❐ pay intervals (hourly, weekly, monthly)
❐ hours of work – including overtime
❐ holiday entitlement including Public Holidays
❐ job title or job description
❐ place of work
❐ sickness and injury rules
❐ pension scheme
❐ length of notice – for both employer and employee
❐ disciplinary rules
❐ grievance procedure including named person.

Specimen statements of employment can be obtained from the Department for Education and Employment or suitable blank written contracts purchased from a stationer. Once prepared the statement or contract should be signed by both parties and the employee should be given a copy to keep. Any changes in employment must be notified in writing within one month of being instituted.

Race discrimination

The Race Relations Act 1976 makes it unlawful for an employer in Great Britain to discriminate against a person of a particular racial group on the grounds of colour, race, nationality or ethnic origins.

It is unlawful to publish an advertisement which indicates an intention by any person to discriminate, regardless of whether such action would be lawful or unlawful.

Direct discrimination is where on racial grounds alone, a person is treated less favourably than others. Indirect discrimination is where a requirement or condition applies with which a small racial group could not comply and is not justifiable and is to the detriment of that person because he or she cannot comply with it, for example an advertisement for a veterinary assistant in a Christian practice could imply that there was discrimination against non-Christians.

With job applications an employer must not discriminate in the terms on which he offers an applicant a job or by refusing to consider an application or by deliberately neglecting to offer the applicant a job.

Sex discrimination and equal pay

The Sex Discrimination Act 1975 (as amended) makes it unlawful for an employer to discriminate against a person on the grounds of his or her sex. This extends to recruitment (including the wording of an advertisement), terms and conditions of employment, access to training, opportunities for promotion and benefits and facilities, and to retirement and dismissal. Discrimination in employment against a married person (of either sex) on the grounds of marital status, is also an offence.

The Equal Pay Act 1970 provides that it is unlawful to discriminate between men and women in regard to pay and in the terms of their contracts of employment (overtime, bonus, holiday and sick leave, etc.). This also includes part-time employees.

A woman must not be employed on less favourable terms and conditions than a man if the work she is doing is the same, or broadly similar, to the work done by a man employed within Great Britain. An exception is treatment afforded to a woman in connection with the birth, or expected birth, of a child. It is unlawful for a firm to discriminate against a woman when taking on a new partner, i.e. in the terms in which she is offered a partnership or by refusing, or deliberately neglecting to offer her a partnership.

The Sex Discrimination Act does not specifically mention harassment but there are specific recommendations and a Code of Practice from the European Commission on measures to combat sexual harassment, which can apply if during their employment an individual is subject to verbal, non-verbal or physical conduct on the basis of their sex or marital status, which they clearly do not want or welcome. It is also possible that failure by an employer to deal with such conduct could constitute discrimination.

Disabled workers

The Disability Discrimination Act 1995 makes it unlawful to 'unjustifiably' discriminate against an individual on the grounds of his or her disability in relation to recruitment, training, benefits, terms and conditions of employment and dismissal.

All employers of 20 employees or more have a statutory obligation to employ a quota (currently 3%) of registered disabled workers for a period of 30 hours per week (which counts as a full unit). If insufficient numbers of registered disabled persons cannot be found to fill the quota an employer may apply for a permit enabling employment of persons not registered as disabled.

Statutory sick pay (SSP)

Employers now have to take on the responsibility for the payment of sick pay to their employees. The Statutory Sick Pay Act 1994 removed the right of employees to reclaim from the government payments properly made by deductions from NI Contributions. An SSP compensation scheme called the New Relief Scheme (NRS) helps all employers faced with exceptionally high levels of sickness pay. This scheme provides for full reimbursement of an employer's costs paid in any month when they exceed 13% of the employer's gross National Insurance contributions (employers and employees) for that month.

All statutory sick pay payments to employees count as earnings and are subject to the normal PAYE and National Insurance contributions. The employee has to first have a period of incapacity for work (PIW) which means an absence from work of four consecutive days (these need not necessarily all be working days). Once a PIW exists there is a period of entitlement to qualifying days: however the first three qualifying days in a period of entitlement are 'waiting days' and do not qualify for sick pay. All eligible employees are entitled to only one standard rate of SSP, which at the time of writing is £60.20 a week. No SSP is payable where the weekly earnings are less than £67.00.

Incapacity benefit

There is a maximum period of 28 weeks of payment of SSP after which the employee must claim an incapacity benefit allowance direct from the DSS and be subject to an independent medical examination from a doctor appointed by the Benefits Agency to assess whether they are capable of work and this is not just the job that they were employed to carry out, but any kind of work. Incapacity benefits payments will cease (subject to limited exceptions) if the individual is assessed as being fit for some kind of work, e.g. a car park attendant.

Maternity rights

The following minimum rights have been agreed under the EU Pregnant Workers Directive.

❐ Fourteen weeks continuous leave allocated before/after childbirth.
❐ Paid time off for antenatal examinations.
❐ No dismissal during the period of pregnancy and maternity leave.
❐ Contractual rights preserved during maternity leave.
❐ Pay at a rate not less than the appropriate sick pay during period of maternity.

In the UK all women, irrespective of length of service and number of hours worked will be entitled to a minimum of 14 weeks maternity leave. This basic maternity leave may commence at any time the woman wishes after the 11th week before the expected week of childbirth (EWC).

Her contract of employment continues during this basic leave and the employer must maintain all contractual benefits such as private health insurance, company car for private use, the accrual of holiday entitlement. The exception is remuneration, which during basic leave is specifically excluded. The mother has a right to return to work at any time before the end of 29 weeks beginning with the week in which the birth occurred, provided that she notifies her employer in writing 21 days in advance of her intended date of return.

On her return to work she must be reinstated in the same kind of job as before and on terms and conditions not less favourable than she enjoyed before. However, if the business employs five or fewer people she loses her right to return to work if it is not reasonably practicable for the employer to offer her suitable employment.

Statutory Maternity Pay is payable for a period of up to 18 weeks by employers to employees who have stopped working because of pregnancy or childbirth provided that they have been continuously employed for 26 weeks ending with the 15th week before the expected week of confinement.

Minimum period of notice

However small the business, employees are entitled to a minimum of one week's notice after four weeks' continuous employment. After two years their entitlement increases to one week's notice for each year of service to a maximum of 12 weeks' notice.

Payment in lieu of notice can be offered as an alternative to cover the period required by legislation. The employer may agree a contract which includes longer periods of notice. These minimum rights do not apply if the employee is dismissed for gross misconduct.

Dismissal

Any employee with job security under the employment legislation should only be dismissed in accord with the current legislation and within the terms of any contract of employment. They have a right not to be unfairly dismissed and if they consider that it was unfair, they can present a complaint to an employment tribunal.

Fair reasons for dismissal must be based on:

❏ employee's capability or qualification to perform work (this includes employee's health)
❏ employee's conduct
❏ redundancy
❏ employee cannot continue working without breaking the law
❏ other substantial reasons such as personality conflicts, business reorganisations.

There must also be fair procedures for dismissal. Employees should rarely be dismissed for a first offence and the employer must be able to show that in all the circumstances, including the size of the business and its administrative resources, he acted fairly and reasonably in treating the facts as a basis for dismissal.

The employee should be given a formal verbal warning; this should be followed by a written warning setting out the likely consequences of further offences and an opportunity to explain themselves. Further misconduct will result in a final written warning stating that a reoccurrence of the offence is likely to lead to suspension or dismissal.

Gross misconduct, such as persistent drunkenness on the job, wilful refusal to follow lawful and reasonable orders, dishonesty, physical attack on other staff, gross neglect and breach of safety rules may justify instant dismissal but there is usually time and justification for a warning before action.

Placing an employee in an untenable position, thus compelling him or her to resign is called constructive dismissal and may amount to unfair dismissal and is usually a breach of the contract of employment. If you can lawfully dismiss, you must give the statutory notice and written reasons for your action should be sent to the employee within 14 days of the dismissal.

When the dismissal is unfair the employee is entitled to reinstatement in the same job or re-engagement in a similar job and an additional compensation award. He or she can claim compensation by agreement or via the employment tribunal. The basic award is related to the actual financial loss by reference to the period plus the amount of any benefit the employee might reasonably have expected to receive from the job plus a compensatory award which had a maximum in 1999 of £12 000.

Exclusions from the unfair dismissal procedures are as follows.

❑ An employee who has not been continuously employed by the employer for one year. (This does not apply if the dismissal is on grounds of unlawful racial or sex discrimination.)
❑ Employees who have reached the normal age of retirement.
❑ Employees who under the contract of employment normally work outside Great Britain.
❑ Fixed term contracts of one year or more which have specified in writing to exclude any claim for unfair dismissal.

An additional award may be made if an order for reinstatement or reengagement is made and the terms of the order are not fully complied with. A special award may also be made as compensation for employees who have been dismissed on grounds of their union membership or activities.

Part-time workers

Part-time workers are now entitled to the same statutory rights as full-time employees. Employees still need to be in employment for a certain time before qualifying for these statutory rights. For example everyone, regardless of how many hours worked, now needs one year's continuous service to gain rights to claim unfair dismissal.

Transfer of undertakings

The Transfer of Undertakings Regulations 1981 apply in cases where a business is transferred from one owner to another, whether by sale or on death of the owner. This applies whether the owner is an individual, a partnership or a limited company.

Where such a transfer takes place the new employer is required to observe all the terms and conditions of employment that applied to the employees before the transfer – except for occupational pension schemes. If a fundamental change to the contract is made as a result of the transfer, the employee may leave and claim constructive dismissal. It would then be for the employer to show that there was a good reason for the change and that it had been introduced in a fair manner.

An employee who was dismissed either before or after such a transfer is treated as being unfairly dismissed unless it can be shown that there was an economic, technical or organisational reason for the changes in the workforce and this was the principal reason for the dismissal. In that case, the fairness of the dismissal would be tested under the normal unfair dismissal rules.

Redundancy

Under the Redundancy Payments Act 1965, an employee with two years' continuous service who is made redundant can claim redundancy payments. The amount of redundancy pay depends on the employee's age and length of employment and ranges from half a week's pay to one and a half weeks' pay for each year of continuous employment.

There is a maximum payment for 20 years employment and earnings above £220 a week will not be taken into account. In 1999 this represented a maximum payment of £6600. Employment up to the age of 18 years does not count nor does employment over the age of 65.

Unfair redundancy may result in unfair dismissal claims. A common complaint is that the employee was unfairly selected for redundancy because the formula of 'last in, first out' has not been followed or that the manner of implementing the redundancy was unfair. If the employees are members of an independent trade union, both sides are well advised to consult with their representatives before implementing redundancy action. Large organisations must consult with trade unions before making redundancies.

In the case of a change of ownership of a practice, where an employee continues to work for the new owner, the employee is not entitled to any redundancy pay, but in the event of redundancy occurring at a later date the payment (to be made entirely by the new owner) will then be based on the whole of the employee's continuous service under the previous and the new owner.

Employees will not be entitled to redundancy payments if they unreasonably refuse an offer by the new owner, either to be re-engaged on the same terms without a break in their employment or to be re-engaged on different terms provided the offer is made in writing before the change of ownership takes place and the offer is suitable in relation to the employee.

In the case of the death of an employer, when the business is carried on by his personal representative and the employees agree to be re-engaged within eight weeks after the employer's death, they are not entitled to any redundancy pay.

The national minimum wage

All workers in the UK now have a legal right to a minimum level of pay which is the national minimum wage. This became law on 1 April 1999 and applies to both full time and part time workers.

The minimum hourly rate in October 2000 for 18–21 year olds is £3.20 and for 22 year olds and above is £3.70. The minimum wage does not apply to under 18s or to trainees who do not work under a contract of employment. Provision of the benefit of accommodation can allow for 50p an hour to be deducted from the minimum wage.

Non-compliance with the minimum wage is a serious offence and an enforcement body has been set up to deal with complaints, which can be taken before an employment tribunal.

The working time regulations

These regulations came into force in October 1998 and implement the European Working Time Directive for workers above the minimum age of 18.

The basic rights are as follows.

(1) A limit of an average of 48 hours a week which a worker can be required to work. (However this is averaged over a 17-week period. In any case workers can contract out of these regulations and can choose to work more hours if they want to.)

(2) A limit of an average of 8 hours work in 24 which night workers can be required to work

(3) A right for night workers to receive free health assessments

(4) A right to 11 hours rest per day

(5) A right to a day off per week

(6) A right to an in-work rest break if the working day is longer than six hours

(7) A right to four weeks paid leave per year

Some sectors are excluded such as road, rail, air, inland waterway and sea fishing. Veterinary practice is NOT an excluded sector.

Time spent by veterinary surgeons and nurses on call, when you are at the disposal of your employer but not carrying out any duties, does not count as working time for the purpose of these regulations.

Further details on recent employment legislation can be obtained from the DTI website (www.dti.gov.uk).

Chapter 38
Limited Companies
John Gripper

Following a decision at the 1997 November Council Meeting, The Royal College of Veterinary Surgeons modified its advice on incorporation and acknowledged that the College has no legal powers to prevent members from forming a company for the ownership and management of a veterinary practice.

There is now no restriction on the ownership of a veterinary practice, which can be owned by a limited company (provided that the directors are not disqualified under company law) or any private individual who does not need to have any veterinary qualifications. It is now also possible for a veterinary surgeon to form a veterinary partnership with a person who is not a qualified veterinarian.

It has always been possible to form a service company alongside a partnership provided the service company did not practice veterinary surgery, however this new advice from the College means that the ownership and control of veterinary practices can now pass out of the hands of the profession.

The arrival of pet superstores and their 'look-alikes' with the opening of in-store veterinary clinics has resurrected the debate on the issue of veterinary practices forming limited companies. At the same time there has been the announcement in the financial press that KPMG, one of the largest accountancy firms, is planning to incorporate its audit work in order to shield itself from high professional negligence claims.

Advantages

The advantages of a limited company can be divided into three main groups:

Limited liability
Because a company is a separate legal entity, any amounts owing in a liquidation can only be offset against the assets of the company itself unless the directors have pledged their own assets as security. However, because a claim for professional negligence may be made against the individual veterinary surgeon in a personal capacity, it may be necessary to consider personal insurance cover.

Apart from a few veterinary practices treating high value single animals such as a thoroughbred stallion, the veterinary profession does not have difficulty in obtaining professional indemnity at reasonable rates. This compares favourably to other professions such as solicitors and accountants where costs tend to be very much higher, although the nature of the risk may be rather different.

It would damage the image of the veterinary profession to shelter behind the artificial protection of company limited liability. The Royal College of Veterinary Surgeons has now decided that it should be mandatory for all veterinary practices to have full insurance cover for professional negligence.

It would therefore appear that the formation of a limited company would not be advantageous as a method of limiting the liability of practitioners in veterinary practice.

The Limited Liability Partnership Act 2000 is a hybrid between a limited company and a partnership, enabling partners to benefit from limited liability status. There is however still a potential claim against the individual in tort law, rather than contract.

Tax benefits

The rate of corporation tax for small companies starts at 10% for the first £10 000 of profit after charging all costs including directors' salaries; it is then taxed at 20% (on a marginal relief basis up to £50 000 and thereafter at 20% up to £1 500 000). The main rate is 30%. The directors can take out money as either dividends or salary. The main advantage of dividends is that no National Insurance is payable so that a director can receive a salary up to the higher tax rate thresholds and then the remainder of his profit can be paid as dividends. If profits are retained within the business, then using a company may produce a cash flow advantage because of the lower corporation tax rates.

There is therefore a potential tax advantage for the partner who is a substantial higher rate taxpayer at 40%. In a partnership income tax is payable on the whole of the profit share, whether it is drawn out or not.

In the company profit that is retained in the business will only be taxed at corporation tax level (20%) as compared to the higher rate of personal income tax in a partnership. However, if a partner has high personal expenditure requiring withdrawal of the full profit share, no advantage will occur.

A company director can obtain more generous pension arrangements than a self-employed partner. Also it is easier to obtain better terms for HP/leasing on expensive equipment for a limited company. The raising of capital finance becomes easier because there is an opportunity within a company for outside shareholders to invest capital in the business. In some other professions they insist that 75% control must remain with the professional directors.

Corporate structure and staffing

One of the main advantages with a corporate structure is that there is greater flexibility for bringing younger members of the profession into the business as directors without the need to insist on large capital inputs. Likewise staff could move on after a period without the long-term commitment of a partnership where dissolution can be fraught with difficulties.

It was felt that this greater flexibility of personal mobility would be of particular benefit to the increasing number of young female veterinary surgeons who are often reluctant to make long-term commitments.

Within the company structure it is easier to introduce a profit sharing scheme and encourage a 'team' attitude. There is the option of offering staff a shareholding or inviting them to become stakeholders (to coin a phrase).

Disadvantages

(1) The accounts of a limited company have to be audited and placed on public record, if the turnover exceeds £1 million and the balance sheet total exceeds £1.4 million. Prior to 26 July 2000 the turnover limit was £350 000.

(2) Setting up a company involves substantial initial costs for professional advice, stamp duty, purchase of a company, change of stationery, etc. These costs have been estimated at about £5000 for a large practice.

(3) There are tax consequences in the timing of the transfer of a partnership into a limited company such as cessation provisions, rollover of capital gains tax and VAT in respect of transfer of undertaking rules.

(4) Consideration will need to be given as to whether it is advisable or not to transfer partnership properties into the limited company.

It seems that for the majority of veterinary practices the disadvantages may outweigh the advantages but for the larger veterinary practice and the more profitable practices where the principal or partner is earning a high income (£75K plus) then it may be beneficial to consider a change.

The decision as to whether to change to a limited liability company is very dependent on the personal and financial circumstances of the individual partners and very detailed analysis and full debate should take place with your legal and financial advisors before any decision is made.

Chapter 39
Buying and Selling a Partnership
Dixon Gunn

The buying and selling of partnerships are separate parts of practice ownership and the aims of the individual at each stage must be recognised. Buying is more difficult because of the capital investment to be made. Selling usually takes place at a time when the outgoing partner has time to evaluate his personal finance and decide when to retire.

In this chapter the valuation of the practice is presumed to have taken place and here we discuss the methods of buying in, or being bought out. The starting point is the list of assets and this list is found in the balance sheet of the practice accounts. As has often been said, the balance sheet is much more important than the profit and loss account, which only states how much has been earned in total and how much is left after the accountant has deducted all the allowable expenses of the practice.

If you are inviting someone to join you or you have been invited to join a practice, the balance sheet is the prime document to look at. And this is where buying in differs from selling, because you do not have to use the whole balance sheet if buying in, whereas you will more than likely want to use it if retiring.

Consider a list of practice assets as seen in the average balance sheet and identify those which are to be included in any purchase or sale.

The assets are:

❏ Property
 – Owned
 – Leased

❏ Veterinary equipment
 – Owned
 – Leased
 – Hire purchase

❏ Office equipment
 – Owned
 – Leased
 – Hire purchase

❏ Household equipment
 – Usually owned

❏ Investments and prepayments

❏ Drugs in stock

❏ Motor vehicles
 – Owned
 – Leased
 – Hire purchase

❏   Goodwill or equivalent

❏   Debtors and creditors

❏   Cash at bank and in hand

The incoming partner will definitely be involved with the first six items and if the cars are owned by the practice, these as well. Goodwill, debtors and creditors and cash at bank are optional for a purchase.

For a retirement, the whole list is part of the practice and must be considered. Each item on the list of assets must be considered separately.

Property

This can be freehold or leased property and in this context 'leased' is relatively short-term, i.e. 25 years or less. Partners buying in should pay for their share of this property and indeed their share of the lease. But what if the property is worth £150 000 and the mortgage is £100 000? There is no way that the incoming partner should pay for a share of £150 000 and still be responsible for part of the £100 000 mortgage. So a valuation of the property must discount the outstanding mortgage and then the practice must make sure that the source of finance, the company lending the money, knows that a change in percentage ownership has taken place. This type of arrangement immediately involves 'financial creditors' because the outstanding mortgage acts as a creditor, i.e. one to whom you owe money.

If you are buying in, buy a share of the property or a share in the lease and if the property is not all paid for, buy a share of the debt, which reduces the input you have to make. The simplest route to follow is the one in which all the partners own all the property in the same percentage share as their ownership of the practice.

In some cases the property is definitely not for sale and the partnership must become a tenant of the owners. A lease detailing all the arrangements must be drawn up so that the partnership has the security of being the legal tenant. It is also wise to include an option to purchase should the owner(s) decide to sell. This arrangement has capital gains tax disadvantages for partners who are also owners, which must not be ignored.

Veterinary equipment

Veterinary equipment is either owned or leased or on lease/hire purchase. The problem comes with a leasing company being involved and the detail of the lease. Is it a lease purchase, so that it is owned at the end of the lease period? Is it a perpetual lease and never owned? If it is a perpetual lease, then as the incoming partner, there is nothing to buy, but there is a share of the leasing costs to be paid in future.

If the article is on a lease/hire purchase agreement, the figure to pay will depend on the years left for payment and the purchase price at the end of that time. As an example an X-ray set may be lease purchased over five years. After five years the purchase is a nominal £10. The second hand value of the set is £2500. Leasing costs still to be paid are £2400 and there is the £10 to pay as the peppercorn purchase. The value of taking over the lease is £90 for the whole practice – £2500 of the current value minus £2410 made up from £2400 of leasing costs still to pay and the £10 purchase price at the end of the leasing period.

When valuing equipment make sure the leasing or hire purchase arrangements in force at the time are examined closely. It is in fact a criminal offence to sell an article that is not owned because of a lease or hire purchase agreement.

Office and household equipment

Office equipment, for example typewriters and filing cabinets and household equipment, such as washing machines, refrigerators, kettles, cookers, settees and the like should be dealt with in exactly the same way as veterinary equipment.

This is often an extensive list with computers forming a major item. Take care that the ownership is clearly defined before a share is bought or sold.

Investments and prepayments

An example of investments are shares in a veterinary wholesale company paid for by the practice. Prepayments are payments for items such as insurance and car road tax where a whole year is paid for in advance and part of this time overlaps the transfer of ownership. It is therefore quite fair to have to buy a share or sell a share on retiring. The figure usually presented by the practice accountant is simple to calculate.

Drugs in stock

This should be a simple subject but current purchasing arrangements do complicate it. The actual value of stock in hand at the time of purchase or sale of a share should be determined by listing all unopened containers and untapped bottles of in-date stock on the shelves and in the cars at the appropriate date. The purchase face price should be applied to this list to value the stock in hand. In any active practice there will be a considerable number of tapped bottles and opened containers, which are 'gained' by the purchaser and 'lost' to the vendor.

The purchase face price is not necessarily what the practice has paid for the stock in hand. There are prompt settlement discounts, retrospective discounts and bulk purchase discounts. Of these only the prompt settlement discount will apply to most of the stock in hand. Either the discount can be taken to equate with all the opened containers and bottles which have not been included in the price, or an agreed discount on face price can be negotiated.

Retrospective discounts, which may be received after the alteration in the partnership, must be considered carefully to determine the period of purchase to which they apply. Depending on the timing, they belong either to the 'old' partnership or the 'new'. Bulk purchase discounts usually received directly from the pharmaceutical company are more specific and can be attributed to stock in hand if still on the shelf. An adjustment to value of the stock can be made if necessary.

Motor vehicles

Cars can be owned by the practice, privately owned by partners, leased, on hire purchase or contract hire.

Buying or selling only arises when the practice owns the car or is buying it by means of a deferred payment system. Again the true position must be established and the companies involved informed of any change in the arrangements. If the car is being bought on hire purchase, then the outstanding payments must be deducted from the current value to determine the value of the car for the incoming or outgoing partner.

Goodwill or equivalent

If goodwill is still included as a capital asset of the practice it will be valued according to the current arrangements within the practice and the sum either paid in by the purchaser or paid out to the retiring partner. A lump sum in the hands of the retiring partner might be liable to capital gains tax.

An alternative method is to write out goodwill from the practice so that the purchaser does not pay a lump sum nor does the retiring partner receive one. However, the retiring partner can receive a pension paid by the practice for a period of years and a new partner has to be responsible for his share of such pensions. The pension is liable to income tax in the hands of the retired partner but the cost of it is allowable as a practice expense.

Depending on the age of the partners, a system of graded distribution of net profits (GDNP) between partners can be established which allows all partners in turn to invest in their personal pension funds, at the expense of their juniors. On retirement they do not receive a capital payment for goodwill, or a pension from the practice; they do, however, have a life-long pension from the company or companies of their choice in effect paid for by their partners (see Chapters 15 and 34).

Debtors and creditors, cash at bank and in hand

Consider two similar practices except that Practice B has taken out a loan (see Table 39.1).

Table 39.1 Comparison of Practice A and Practice B assets and liabilities.

	Practice A	Practice B
	(£)	(£)
Assets		
Debtors	30,000	30,000
Bank balance and cash in hand	21,000	21,000
	51,000	51,000
Liabilities		
Creditors	16,000	16,000
VAT account	5,000	5,000
Loan	–	60,000
	21,000	81,000
Net assets (liabilities)	30,000	(30,000)

Practice A

If a young veterinary surgeon is buying into a third of practice A, he or she has to find an additional £10 000 (a third of £30 000 of net assets) to join in and this £10 000 is a personal cost, to be repaid with interest. It is possible to leave these assets with the *in situ* partners; they can collect the debts, pay the bills and in theory divide the £30 000 between them at the end of the day. The new practice is of course without funds to start with and an agreed overdraft with the bank must be arranged. This is not difficult because of the history of the previous practice. This method does mean that two accounts must be run in parallel until the 'old' practice has collected in all the money owed and paid all its bills.

A simpler way of reducing the sum to be paid by the incoming partner is for the existing partners to make an additional drawing of £21 000, the sum of the cash held by the practice. This has the effect of reducing net assets to £9000 and the sum to be found by the incoming partner is now £3000. In this case there is no need to run parallel accounts.

Practice B

If however, the assets remain the same as before, but liabilities are increased by a loan of £60 000 to a total of £81 000 as in Practice B, then net assets become net liabilities of £30 000. This actually decreases the value of the practice and of course should be involved in the final calculation for the incoming partner, reducing the sum to be paid by £10 000 for a third share of the total practice asset. He is, in addition, responsible for his share of the loan.

Retirement

Debtors and creditors obviously have to be included in the calculation when a partner retires. He has to pay his share of the agreed list of debts. There may be an item or two under dispute, for example £1000 held over on the failure to make good a terrazzo floor. The retiring partner has to decide whether or not he will leave money in to cover this or pay up if the practice ever has to pay.

Debtors in mixed or large animal practice are more of a problem. The practice will not receive all the money owed. A negotiation with the continuing partners is essential. The practice should write off all likely bad debts and only pay out on the net sum. The retired partner can be paid his share of unexpectedly recovered debts as and when they are received.

Contracts of partnership usually do, and indeed should, dictate how the retiring partner should be paid, e.g. a quarter every three months or six months with interest on the outstanding sum at 1% to 2% over bank base rate. That is simple. What is better is to leave as little in the retiring partner's capital account as possible at the point of retirement and the way for the retiring partner to achieve this is, with his partners' permission, to grossly overdraw during the last years of his involvement. In a multiman practice the ongoing partners should realise they have got to pay him out and payment by this method is reasonably painless. By restricting their drawings a little, cash flow should not be disturbed overmuch.

There is one other aspect of taking in a new partner that is worthy of consideration. The question to put is 'Does the practice really need the money just now?' Surprisingly the answer is not always 'Yes'.

Say for simplicity that the total value of the assets to be transferred in a partnership moving from two to three partners is £150 000. The two established partners have £75 000 each in their partners' accounts. In theory the newcomer should produce £50 000 and the two older partners remove £25 000 each and they all end up with £50 000 each in their new capital accounts.

If borrowing £50 000 is difficult for the incoming partner, then he or she can put in £30 000 instead. The effect on the capital accounts is as shown in Table 39.2. This does not mean that the partners are not equal partners in terms of sharing net profit. They are legally equal partners, but the new

Table 39.2 The effect on capital accounts of borrowing £50,000 or £30,000.

Partners:	A	B	C	Total
Existing capital	75,000	75,000		150,000
Full payment introduced			50,000	50,000
withdrawn	25,000	25,000		(50,000)
	50,000	50,000	50,000	150,000
Existing capital	75,000	75,000		150,000
Part payment introduced			30,000	30,000
withdrawn	15,000	15,000		(30,000)
	60,000	60,000	30,000	150,000

partner has not paid for his whole share. He is borrowing £20 000 from his partners and he has to pay for that. It is a very nice place to borrow from because there is no security requested and there are no repayment terms set down.

The two senior partners are capitalising the practice by £30 000 each more than their equal partner, so they must receive interest on this £30 000 before profits are divided. Interest can be set at $X\%$ above base rate at the midpoint in the practice year. Then at the year end they receive their 'interest on capital' before dividing the profits. Over a number of years, by dint of the new partner paying less tax and by restricting drawings as much as possible, the three accounts can grow together. This is discussed in greater detail in Chapter 40. It is a helpful method to aid the introduction of the right person into what should be a mutually supportive group of persons – the partnership.

Chapter 40

Payment by the Incoming Partner

Dixon Gunn

In Chapter 39 I briefly mentioned alternative methods of paying for goodwill. This chapter discusses how an incoming partner may pay for all the assets of the practice.

Capital input versus share

It is important to understand that there is no fixed relationship between the capital invested in a practice by a partner and that partner's right to receive a certain percentage of net profits. A partner can quite legitimately have 80% of the value of the practice credited to his name and still be content to receive 20% of the net profit.

Partners must learn to distinguish between their capital investment and the way in which the net profits are divided. They are in fact unrelated. At its simplest in a 50:50 partnership two partners will have equal sums invested and share net profits equally. But even in this simplest of scenarios, the sums invested will vary.

Partnership accounts

The sum invested by a partner is the capital in his partnership account. This can be identified in one account simply called 'Partner's Account' or in two accounts commonly called 'Capital Account' and 'Current Account'. There is in fact little reason to have two accounts per partner. The capital account is seen as representing investment in bricks and mortar and does not change from year to year unless the partners decide to revalue the property. The current account takes care of the spending money. Net profit share is added in and drawings including tax and NI are taken out. Because of variation in tax allowances, insurance premiums and drawings, the current accounts will never stay exactly equal. They can be equalised by one partner taking a final drawing at the end of the year to realign accounts. Complications can arise when, for example, a revaluation of property is shared between the partners and the adjustment up or down is included, quite wrongly, in the current account.

But what of an adjustment to the value of equipment, when a new partner joins? Is this capital account or current account? The fact of having two accounts becomes significant when the partners have agreed that there will be an interest payment made to partners for sums invested. Will this be on the capital account, on the current account or on both? If the decision is to opt for the capital account only, then a shrewd partner in an unsuspecting practice could overdraw his current account without penalty.

Interest payments, discussed below, should be based on the total investment of each partner, that is the sum of his capital and current account, or more appropriately on his 'account' representing his total investment.

Assets to be paid for

As discussed in Chapter 39 the assets involved can be identified as property, equipment, stock, motor vehicles and goodwill with an adjustment for financial assets less liabilities.

This list splits into two parts, with goodwill on one side and all the other assets on the other side. The major list of all the assets less liabilities will have a finite value and these will be identified in the opening balance sheet of the new partnership. The new partner can be expected to have to find the capital to invest in these assets. The goodwill value of the practice may not be recorded in the balance sheet and there is no need to include it. The method of payment for this intangible asset should reflect the fact that it is not a defined asset of the business.

Methods of payment

There are three methods of payment: the first two are capable of being used for all the assets, the third is more applicable to goodwill.

Capital payment in total
This first method is simple and sometimes difficult for the incoming partner. It is quite simply 'pay into the practice the capital sum due for your share'.

If the incoming partner is able to do this, what then happens to this money? Is it left in to support the practice or is it withdrawn immediately by the vendor partner(s)?

Two short scenarios are set out below:

Principal selling an equal share to an incoming partner

Example 1

	Principal	New Partner	Total
	(£)	(£)	(£)
Accounts as at 31/12/X	100,000	–	100,000
Capital introduced	–	50,000	50,000
Drawings	(50,000)	–	(50,000)
Partners' accounts	50,000	50,000	100,000

Example 2

	Principal	New Partner	Total
	(£)	(£)	(£)
Accounts as at 31/12/X	100,000	–	100,000
Capital introduced	–	50,000	50,000
Drawings	(25,000)	–	(25,000)
Partners' accounts	75,000	50,000	125,000

In Example 1 the partners' accounts stay equal and no action is required. In Example 2, because the principal has only withdrawn half of the introduced capital, the value of the balance sheet of the practice has been increased, presumably by reducing a practice overdraft or loan by £25 000. The new position is that one partner is financing the practice to a greater extent than the other partner. He deserves a reward for this by way of an interest payment. The method of determining this payment is discussed below, because it becomes of even greater importance in discussing the second method of payment, partial capital payment.

Partial capital payment

In many practices, the sum to be paid by the incoming partner can impose severe difficulties on the individual in terms of raising the capital because of his/her personal commitments, for example a house mortgage. The forecast profits of the practice may not meet the requirements of the financial institution lending the money. This latter consideration can be due to the current financial situation of the country as a whole and not the practice in insularity.

In this case, the established practice may say to the incoming partner 'You should pay in £50 000 but we will accept a lesser payment of £30 000 and adjust our partner accounts accordingly'. The two-person practice scenarios of Examples 1 and 2 are now used to show the new scenario (Example 3):

Example 3

	Principal	New Partner	Total
	(£)	(£)	(£)
Accounts as at 31/12/X	100,000	–	100,000
Capital introduced	–	30,000	30,000
Drawings	(30,000)	–	(30,000)
Partners' accounts	70,000	30,000	100,000

Once again one partner is financing the practice to a greater extent than the other. This could be made worse by the principal withdrawing less than the new partner has introduced, as in Example 2 above. The gap in the accounts has to be bridged by rewarding the partner who is in fact financing the practice. Without this money, the practice would have to arrange additional borrowing.

The method of rewarding partners in this situation is to set up a system of paying interest to partners on their investment. The payment can be based on the excess investment over and above the investment of the other partner(s) or it can be arranged in such a way that each partner receives interest on their investment. Because of the complexities of shares and numbers of partners, this latter method is the simplest. The interest rate to be used has to be agreed. It is commonly linked to bank base rate and expressed as base rate plus $X\%$. As base rates change, the application date must also be selected. Further the date or dates on which the capital in the partner's name is to be measured for the purpose of determining the interest must also be agreed.

A simple but effective formula can be written as follows:

Interest of base rate plus $X\%$ will be paid at the end of the practice year as a prior claim on net profits, on the capital standing to each partner's name on the first day of the financial year. The base rate selected will be that in operation at the midpoint of the practice year.

Payments can be calculated monthly, quarterly, or six-monthly, but for most partnerships a once a year payment should suffice if there is correct control over partners' drawings.

Applying the simple method to Example 3 and taking the interest rate at 10%, then before the net profits are divided, the principal would have £7000 (10% of £70 000) credited to his account and the new partner would have £3000 credited to his/her account.

By dint of taking smaller drawings and very likely having a smaller tax bill to pay, the new partner increases his account year by year until parity is reached. This is a beneficial way of assisting a new partner to buy into the assets of the business. In effect he borrows from the business and pays it back as and when he can by restricting his drawings.

Graded distribution of net profits (GDNP)

This method of paying for a partnership adopts an entirely different approach to payment for goodwill. Traditionally this was paid for out of capital, which means that income tax had to be paid on the earnings before the remaining capital was passed on. Or more likely, the sum was borrowed and the capital saved after paying income tax is used to repay the borrowing.

The GDNP method eliminates goodwill as such and introduces the concept of accepting less than 50% of net profit for a 50% share of the practice. The advantage to the purchasing partner is that by agreeing to transfer profits, they are not considered as earnings and therefore there is no income tax to pay on the transferred sums. The receiving partner has to accept the transfer as part of his income and is liable to pay tax on this unless he can arrange to pay the sum into his pension policy in which case he will avoid a tax payment.

Not only does the incoming partner benefit from transferring sums pre-tax rather than post-tax, he also benefits by delaying total payment over a number of years. For this reason he can be fairly generous in the sums he agrees to transfer and for the number of years that this will continue. For instance if the principal in our example above had hoped to receive £40 000 for 50% of the goodwill before it was agreed to write out goodwill and substitute a GDNP method, the incoming partner could afford to transfer £6000 p.a. for ten years and still benefit from this method.

Combining methods

A principal agrees to sell half his practice to an incoming partner. The balance sheet of the practice, which does not include goodwill, is valued at £100 000. The incoming partner agrees to pay a premium for the right to enjoy the profits of the practice at the rate of £6000 p.a. for ten years. At the end of the first year, the net profit of the partnership is £120 000. The net profit is divided as follows:

	Principal	New Partner	Total
	(£)	(£)	(£)
A. Interest on capital invested	7,000	3,000	10,000
B. Equal shares of net profit	55,000	55,000	110,000
C. GDNP Transfer	6,000	(6,000)	–
Credited to Account	68,000	52,000	120,000

From the sum of £52 000 the new partner has to finance the borrowing of £30 000, the capital he introduced. The reduction in the principal's net profit is not as severe as he might have feared and hopefully a mutually beneficial partnership is created.

Chapter 41
Valuation of Goodwill

John Gripper

When you purchase any business that is a profit making concern, it is standard practice to pay for the goodwill element of that business. The value of the goodwill in a veterinary practice is the sum that you will have to pay over and above the cost of the assets (the property, fittings and fixtures, instruments and equipment and the drugs) in order to buy the business or take a partnership share. The purchase of goodwill gives you a share in an existing business with an immediate continuing income. The alternative of 'putting up your plate' is accompanied by a risk of failure and a possible wait of a number of years before the practice becomes fully established and provides an adequate income.

Some professional partnerships claim that they do not charge an incoming partner for goodwill but instead have adopted a pension scheme that favours the senior partners or they may insist on an injection of working capital that carries no possibility of capital increase. An absence of a goodwill payment may be replaced by a differential share of profit or unequal work loads and time off within the practice.

Where there is a purpose-built veterinary premises it is sometimes a condition of the partnership that the junior partners must purchase a share of this property and agree to buy the senior partner's share when he retires. This may turn out to be a 'white elephant' and never likely to show real capital appreciation.

So an element of goodwill exists in most veterinary practices – the difficulty arises in devising a fair method for its valuation. Market forces will always determine a fair commercial price in the end because the only real value of goodwill is what a purchaser is prepared to pay and what a seller is willing to accept.

Methods of valuation

The oldest and traditional way of valuing goodwill is to relate it to turnover. This is a very crude and unreliable method because turnover may be high due to retail sales of veterinary drugs or diets at low profit margins or veterinary work carried out at a low profitability. That method has been replaced because goodwill should be related to profitability and there are three methods that are in general use:

(1) A factor is applied to the average of the last three years' gross profits of the practice. This eliminates the drug costs but it is a crude method only utilised by some insurance companies and lending institutions.

(2)   An average of the last three years' adjusted net profit for the practice
       is multiplied by an appropriate goodwill factor. This is the current
       method recommended by the Society of Practising Veterinary Sur-
       geons in its 1983 Review of Goodwill.
(3)   A calculation is made to determine the 'super' profit of the practice
       on the basis of the last three years' earnings. A capitalised value is
       obtained by multiplication of the 'true' profit by a factor of 5 or 6.
       This is the method favoured in the USA.

Determination of adjusted net profit

A calculation of the adjusted net profit has to be made from the official
practice accounts. Added back to the net profit is the cost of all veterinary
assistants' salaries or locum fees plus the employer's National Insurance
and accommodation costs.

The adding back of all assistants and locum costs will allow a fair
comparison between all veterinary practices irrespective of their partner:
assistant ratio. Any excess salary or pension paid to the partner's spouse
should also be added back. The determination of an excess will depend on
the real market value of the work undertaken over and above the level of
the minimum National Insurance contribution base figure and after
allowing 10% of this figure for pension premiums. Any partner's personal
expenses that may have been paid by the practice should also be added
back.

All the financial charges which relate to interest paid on mortgages,
loans, overdrafts, hire purchase charges should also be added back, but
not bank charges. This is necessary because it is not a practical possibility
to determine personal loan expenses in some practices where the business
has been used to fund the owner's own private financial requirements. By
adding back all the financial interest charges every practice is put on an
equal footing to establish a true profitability, and it will be up to the new
owner to determine his own borrowing arrangements.

There are also circumstances where a figure has been shown for repairs
and renewals. Sometimes these improvements have been carried out in
excess of the normal likely expenditure on routine annual maintenance.
An adjustment can be made by adding back this excess figure as a non-
recurring expense on freehold property.

A deduction has to be made for a notional rent and no rent has been
shown in the past in the profit and loss accounts, or where there has been
an arm's-length agreement not to pay the full value of the market rent.

Any non-practice income which does not directly relate to the activities
of a veterinary practice should also be deducted, for example bank or
building society interest received, or rent from premises. Fees that have
been received from personal appointments that will not continue such as
lecturing, advisory or director's fees should also be deducted.

Calculation of adjusted net profit

An example for a three person mixed practice with two equal partners employing one veterinary assistant is shown in Table 41.1.

Table 41.1 Calculation of adjusted net profit for a three person mixed practice (two partners and one assistant).

Year ending 30 April	1998	1999	2000
	(£)	(£)	(£)
Turnover	245,000	288,000	310,000
Net profit	82,000	93,000	104,000
Assistant's salary	21,000	22,500	23,500
Assistant's NI	2,142	2,295	2,397
Assistant's accommodation	4,000	4,500	4,500
Locum fees	5,300	2,850	6,700
Excess wives' payments	3,000	4,000	4,000
Excess repairs	9,000	–	–
Overdraft interest	7,800	8,900	4,600
Less notional rent	(10,000)	(10,000)	(10,000)
Less interest received	(1,300)	(1,078)	(456)
Less rent from flat	(3,000)	(2,000)	–
Adjusted net profit	119,942	124,967	139,241
Total adjusted net profit	384,150		
Average adjusted net profit	128,050		

Goodwill factor

The goodwill factor has to be determined for each individual veterinary practice either by agreement within the practice or by an independent valuation. If a valuation is undertaken this can only be carried out by a visit to the practice and the valuer must acquire a full knowledge and have a detailed understanding of all the many different aspects of the individual practice which can affect the goodwill factor such as:

❐ type of practice, i.e. species treated
❐ future growth and profit potential
❐ practice premises, location and parking
❐ geographical, climatic and social conditions affecting travelling
❐ influence of neighbouring practices and charitable animal organisations

❏ willingness of clients to seek veterinary advice
❏ number of veterinary surgeons in practice
❏ ratio of principals and partners to assistants
❏ length of hours worked and time off
❏ level of fees
❏ profitability
❏ debt ratio
❏ income from special appointments
❏ lack of contracts between partners and assistants
❏ special considerations following death of owner
❏ level of drug purchase
❏ return on capital assets
❏ attractiveness of area for staff employment.

After a full and careful consideration of all the above items plus any other special matters that may affect the individual practice a fair assessment of the goodwill factor can then be determined. For the majority of veterinary practices this factor will be between 0.5 and 1.5.

If in our example the goodwill factor was 1.15 then the final calculation for goodwill in the practice would be:

Average adjusted net profit   =   £128 050
Multiplied by goodwill factor of 1.15 =   £147 258

Assistant's discount

If an assistant was buying a share of the goodwill and he had worked in the practice over a period of time and made a contribution to the goodwill then he or she may be entitled to a discount or reduction in the cost of his first share of the goodwill. The Society of Practising Veterinary Surgeons recommends the following scale of discounts as a guideline:

After 1 year   2.5%
       2 years   5%
       3 years   10%
       4 years   15%
       5 years   20%
       6 years   25%
       7 years and above 30%

The time in the practice should be measured to the end of the last financial year used in the calculation of the adjusted net profit for the goodwill valuation.

In the example of an assistant who has worked in the practice for four years, and is joining the partnership with a 30% share, the calculation would be:

	(£)
Total value of goodwill	147,258
30% share	44,177
Less 4 years discount: 15%	(6,627)
Cost of goodwill for assistant	37,550

In this example the assistant's gross income should increase from £23 500 to 38 250 – a three year pay back for the goodwill payment but he or she will have to provide their own house and accept more practice responsibility within the partnership.

However problems can occur in a partnership when a retiring partner is paid out in full for his share of the goodwill, yet the incoming assistant is entering the partnership at a discount to its value. When such a shortfall arises, who is to make up the difference? Is it the outgoing partner or the ongoing partners who lose out?

'Super profit' calculation

A deduction should be made from the net profits at an appropriate 'salary' for the practice principal which is usually related to the cost of employing a veterinary assistant, i.e. $1\frac{1}{2}$ times the cost of a veterinary assistant with two or three years experience.

A deduction may also be made for a management salary in respect of the administration work at 10% of the adjusted net profits and a notional interest charge is deducted for the fixed and liquid assets of the practice. A notional rent may be charged for the property if it is not an asset of the practice.

The net figure of excess earnings or 'true profit' is then capitalised and the value is related to the degree of investment risk involved. This risk has to be evaluated for each practice and could be between a 10% rate (capitalised rate of ten times) or a 20% (capitalised rate of five times).

In our example, averaged over three years:

	(£)
Net profit	93,000
Less partners' salaries	(60,000)
Less management salary	(12,805)
Less interest on assets	(4,000)
Less notional rent	(7,000)
Super profit	9,195
Multiplied by a rate of 5 to 10	= £45,975 to £91,950

The main disadvantage with this method is that with a high capital investment in property and equipment there is often a low return of profitability so that many veterinary practices in the UK have a negative figure when calculated by the super profit method.

Another method of valuation of the entire practice (including goodwill) is use of EBITDA (earnings before interest, tax, depreciation and amortisation). This is used by corporate groups to relate the value of the entire practice as a percentage return on business investment.

Despite predictions to the contrary, there will remain a goodwill value to most veterinary practices for many years to come. However the methods for the calculation of this value will become more sophisticated and so will the alternative methods for the payment of goodwill.

Chapter 42

Partnership Contracts

John Gripper

The definition of a partner is:

> 'A person who has entered into the relationship of partnership i.e. the relationship which subsists between persons carrying on a business in common with a view to profit'.

The Partnership Act 1890 defines business as including every *trade*, *occupation* or *profession*.

In practical terms this means that partners will have a share in both the capital and profits of the business. They also often have joint common tenancy or joint ownership of the property. The partners are jointly and individually liable for the debts of the partnership. Furthermore, unlike a limited company, a partner's liability to meet such debts is not restricted to his capital in the business.

A *salaried partner* who has no direct share in the profits of the business or share in the capital assets is not a true equity holding partner but an employed assistant whose name is held out to the public as a partner. There is a danger that this public declaration of partnership status may make him or her liable to the partnership debts in the same way as the equity partners.

A partnership can exist without a written agreement although this is not advisable as partners fall out, partners become ill and partners die. Memories can fade very quickly as to what was originally agreed when the partnership was first formed.

The Royal College no longer restricts the ownership of veterinary practices to veterinary surgeons, and partnerships can now take place between veterinarians and non-veterinarians such as spouses, investors and other professionals.

The decision to enter a veterinary partnership should not be undertaken lightly – it is just as important as a commitment to get married. In fact a dissolution of partnership can be very similar to divorce – full of acrimony with disagreements about the valuation and distribution of the assets.

Do not enter into a partnership until you have worked together with your prospective partner for a minimum period of a year and have a clear understanding of each other's motivation, ambitions, personal foibles and idiosyncrasies. You should know whether you are going to be compatible working together, without serious personality clashes and have common objectives and aspirations.

The first step when contemplating a partnership is to discuss with each other the broad aspects of the proposed partnership; this should include level of equity and capital holdings, distribution of profits, partnership responsibilities, working arrangements and future retirement plans. Both parties should read the BVA's *Guide to Partnerships in Veterinary Practice*. Each partner should be in agreement over the long-term aims and objectives of the practice and share the same ethical approach. Otherwise differences of opinion and future personality clashes may lie ahead on major policy issues.

Once you have reached general agreement on the broad terms of the partnership, you will then need to arrange for a valuation of the practice assets to be carried out to determine the value of freehold property, goodwill, instruments and equipment, motor cars, debtors and creditors and stock of drugs. You will also need independent financial advice, together with a profit forecast based on current trading, to determine the financial viability of the proposed partnership.

The next stage is to draw up a draft partnership agreement, which will encompass all the points that you have already discussed and reached general agreement on, and present this to the solicitor who will draw up the partnership agreement. When drawing up the final agreement it is advisable for both parties to take independent legal advice from solicitors who have experience in veterinary partnerships.

Arbitration

There should be an arbitration clause in the agreement so that in the event of a dispute between the partners or questions arising out of the interpretation of clauses in the agreement, some independent person such as the President of the RCVS or BVA can appoint an arbitrator.

The appointed arbitrator will not necessarily be a veterinary surgeon, but a member of the Institute of Arbitrators, with appropriate qualifications for carrying out arbitration work. The arbitrator has legal powers and may request an expert in the field to advise him. The arbitrator's decision will be binding on all parties.

Arbitration can be expensive, but taking the dispute to the courts will cost even more. However, disputes within a partnership can be resolved by a mediator who acts as an independent person accepted by both sides, and with experience in dealing with veterinary partnership disputes.

Capital holdings

An incoming partner would normally take a share of the freehold property owned by the partnership; however, the property freeholds can remain in the ownership of the existing partners and be leased to the new partnership or the new partner can take a smaller share of the property assets. The incoming partner may have the option to purchase a further share of the freehold property on the death or retirement of one of the other partners.

The new partnership would take over responsibility for any leasehold property.

It may be agreed that the first share of partnership profits will be divided on the basis of property and other capital holdings as *interest on capital* with the remaining profit divided between the partners on a profit sharing ratio in proportion to their individual equity holdings.

Communication

In all partnerships there should be regular partners' meetings – held at least once a month. These meetings provide an opportunity to discuss all partnership matters, receive the monthly management accounts, deal with staff problems, review each partner's monthly turnover, report on CPD courses and conferences that have been attended and discuss the future growth and direction of the practice in relationship to the business plan.

These should be formal meetings, normally attended by the practice manager; minutes should be taken and all decisions recorded. Many practices find that these meetings are more acceptable if held in the evening on a regular day of the month and combined with some refreshments.

Covenants

Another essential clause in the agreement is one which covers the position if one of the partners leaves, retires or is expelled from the partnership and then proposes to set up again in practice nearby. It is possible to include a clause which will restrict such a person's ability to practise too close, or prevent them from soliciting existing clients. It is important that these covenants are reasonable or the courts will not uphold them. Any restriction put upon retired or expelled partners must not be wider than necessary, either in time or distance or in respect of the type of work which he or she is debarred from carrying out.

Such clauses used to be called 'binding out clauses' or 'restraint of practice'. The subject is dealt with in the *Guide to Veterinary Partnerships in Veterinary Practice* published by the BVA, 7 Mansfield Street, London W1M 0AT.

It is therefore preferable that the practice area is defined by an outline on a map rather than the old 'compass' method, which referred to x miles radius from the main surgery or branch surgery premises. However, the 'compass' method may occasionally still be the most appropriate in some practices.

A restriction period of three to five years is considered reasonable when the retiring partner has been paid out his share of the practice capital (including goodwill) either as a capital sum or as an annuity. If no payment has been made in respect of goodwill then a shorter period may be more appropriate.

It should be made clear to which type of practice or veterinary work any exclusion applies in respect of the retiring partner. To exclude him or her from all kinds of veterinary employment in the area would very likely to be held by the courts to be unduly onerous and the restriction would probably be held void.

It is therefore normally advisable to exclude a partner from only carrying out the work of a veterinary surgeon in general practice that represented the work of the continuing partners e.g. equine or small animal. The exclusion should not prevent the retiring partner from obtaining other types of veterinary employment within the area, which did not represent any competition to the continuing partners.

In order to ensure that a restrictive covenant is given the best chance of being upheld by the courts it is advisable to include a distinct and separate covenant that a retiring or expelled partner will not, for a stated period, act for any client who has been a client of the partnership within the last two years.

Decision making

There is an erroneous view that if a partner holds a slightly larger equity share in the partnership, say 51%, then he or she, as the senior partner, will have a final say in all partnership decisions and can always overrule the junior partner who has only a 49% share.

In a two person practice, where there is a senior and a junior partner with varying capital and equity holdings it may be agreed that, in the case of a disagreement between the partners, then the senior partner shall have greater authority over the junior, but if this is the intention then it *must* be written into the partnership agreement, otherwise each partner has equal voting rights. In a multi-person partnership there may be a clause for majority voting or the agreement may state that if voting is tied, the senior partner may have a casting vote but in order to ensure a harmonious working relationship between the partners it is important that all major decisions are agreed by all the partners.

All the partners, irrespective of their share, must consent to all major partnership decisions, especially those that affect their financial return and the future prospects for the partnership. Examples of a major decision would be the taking in or expulsion of a partner or a major capital commitment to upgrade or build a new practice premises or open a new surgery.

In reaching decisions within the partnership, it should always be remembered that the different ages of each partner will often produce varying viewpoints. The younger partners can take a longer-term view on investments such as the building of a veterinary hospital, which may have only a short-term financial benefit for the older partners. However, the younger partners are often under greater financial pressure through their loans, mortgage and family commitments, and need to maintain a strong income return on their financial investments in the practice.

On the other hand it may be the senior partner who is the driving force in the practice and has the vision and the energy to keep the practice updated with modern buildings, equipment, technology and scientific knowledge.

Dissolution

A dissolution of the partnership may occur by agreement between the partners or by a decision of the arbitrator under the arbitration procedure. Dissolution would also occur in the event of the death of all the partners.

Division of duties

An increasing amount of time has to be spent on the management and administration of a small business such as a veterinary practice. Partners who undertake this responsibility will not be able to spend so much time on clinical fee earning work. This can cause resentment amongst junior partners who believe that the senior partner responsible for practice management may not be 'pulling his weight'. It is only when they themselves become responsible for the management of the practice that they fully realise the importance of a high standard of practice administration in the efficient running of a profitable practice.

Many practices now resolve this situation by the appointment of a practice manager, who will take responsibility for the day to day administration, working within overall policy decisions made by the partners. To be fully effective the practice manager should be regarded as an integral part of the partnership management team.

Another alternative is to divide up the management responsibilities between all the partners so that each partner has his or her own designated area of responsibility i.e. finance, personnel, drugs, duty rotas, motor cars, premises maintenance, fees, laboratory, X-rays and equipment, COSSH, and general administration. At partners' meetings each partner will produce regular reports and recommendations for their particular area of responsibility for approval and ratification by all the partners.

Drawings

A common cause of dispute within a partnership occurs when one partner draws out more than his share of profit and then is either unable or unwilling to refund the excess drawings to the partnership. A clause in the agreement must restrict the amount of drawings to prudent sums agreed between the partners, which allows a reserve for future financial commitments; and the return to the partnership, on request, of any excess drawings by an individual partner.

Duration of partnership

Unless a fixed term of partnership is stated in the partnership agreement then the partnership would continue indefinitely until there is a termination through death or retirement of a partner. In a multi-person partnership it should be made clear that in the event of a retirement of one partner, the partnership will continue between the remaining partners without the need to draw up a new partnership agreement.

In the case of a two-person partnership the death, retirement or expulsion of one partner must end the partnership, because the surviving partner cannot remain in a partnership on his own.

Employment of spouses

Spouses, of either sex, can often be interfering and upset both lay and professional staff, which puts an added strain on relationships within the partnership.

At the start of the partnership the future role and the employment of spouses should be defined and clearly understood so that there will be no recriminations later. Their involvement may be limited to answering the telephone when their spouse is on duty or there may be a bookkeeping position or even a full role as practice manager – all of which should be rewarded by appropriate remuneration.

Expulsion

The partnership agreement will set out the reasons why a partner may be expelled for breach of certain specific actions such as gross misconduct, bankruptcy, insanity or the removal of a partner's name from the Register.

A partner may have his or her name removed from the Register of the Royal College of Veterinary Surgeons for one of the following three reasons:

(1) obtaining Registration by fraudulent means
(2) conviction in the criminal courts of an offence that renders him or her unfit to practise veterinary surgery
(3) disgraceful conduct in a professional respect.

Goodwill

The partnership needs to decide if goodwill is to be included or written out as an asset of the partnership in respect of future changes in the partnership. If goodwill is to be included as an asset then a clear formula or method for the future valuation of goodwill should be written down in the partnership agreement. As the valuation of goodwill will fluctuate according to market circumstances (i.e. the demise of farm practice), it may be preferable just to state that a current goodwill valuation will be determined by an independent valuer who has experience in the valuation of goodwill in veterinary practices.

The agreement should also set out the length of period over which the goodwill will be paid and the interest rate that will apply to any outstanding sum that is due to the retiring partner for both a voluntary and an involuntary retirement, i.e. death, illness or reaching retirement age.

Where goodwill has been written out, the incoming partner may find that he is disadvantaged in other ways in that he may be asked to make contributions to a partners' practice pension scheme, provide alternative working capital, accept a lower share of profit, undertake a higher work load, or have to work additional 'out of hours' rotas to the senior partners.

Holiday and time off duty

The normal holiday arrangements and duty rotas for half days, nights and weekends should be agreed and written down. It is now customary to also include a number of days study leave to attend veterinary meetings, conferences and courses for continuing professional development (CPD)

Problems often occur when some partners want extra time away from the practice to pursue their hobbies or outside interests. Others may want to undertake civic or political activities both within and outside the veterinary profession, i.e. magistrate, local councillor or officer of RCVS, BVA, SPVS or BSAVA. If too much time is spent away from the practice, the absence of the partner may adversely affect the profitability of the practice, although there may be some potential benefits for the practice from the introduction of new ideas, through contacts with other colleagues in the profession.

It is desirable that members should be actively involved in their local community and the affairs of the profession but a fair resolution of their absence from the practice may have to involve the reduction of holiday entitlement or the payment of financial compensation to the other partners for the loss of income that arises from their absence.

Sabbatical leave is becoming more accepted in other professions and it may be decided to include an allowance for sabbatical leave in the agreement.

Incapacity, illness and health

The agreement should set out the length of period for which a partner will receive their full profit share following incapacity resulting in absence from work due to accident or illness. Should the incapacity exceed an agreed length of time, the absent partner will then have to be personally responsible for the payment and associated costs of a locum (accommodation, car and locum agency fees). The agreement should set out the total period of absence from illness, which is allowed before the partnership is terminated.

There are special difficulties when a partner becomes pregnant, especially in the smaller two and three person partnerships. Maternity leave and sick leave are not of course, the same thing. It must be remembered that the other partners will have to work additional duties as a result of the restrictions on the type of work that can be undertaken during pregnancy and the enforced absence from work.

Now that more than half the new veterinary graduates are female, it is important that a clause for maternity leave is included in the partnership agreement which will define the time allowed for maternity leave and the responsibility for the payment of a locum during the absence of the partner from her practice duties. Consideration must now also be given to paternity leave.

Insurance

Cross life assurance between the partners makes sure that in the event of a partner's death, then funds are available so that the remaining partners can pay out the widow(er) or the dependants of the deceased partner. Premiums for life assurance vary according to the age and health of the insured and it is usual for partners to contribute to the premiums of the other partners as they will be receiving the benefits from each other's policies.

The veterinary profession is at the receiving end of an increasing number of claims from a litigious public in respect of alleged professional negligence. The RCVS has now made it mandatory that suitable cover for liability for professional negligence is taken out by the partnership in respect of all veterinary surgeons and staff working in the practice.

Each partner is advised to take out their own permanent accident and sickness cover with the length of benefit waiting period related to the cover provided by the partnership agreement. Consideration should also be given by each partner to critical illness insurance.

Legacies and gifts

There have been instances where grateful clients have made quite substantial personal legacies or gifts to individual veterinary surgeons. This clause clarifies the ownership of such legacies and gifts in relation to the other partners.

It is usual that any legacy or gift not being in direct or express return for professional services rendered made to any partner exclusively shall belong to that partner and shall not be brought into the partnership practice account.

Motor vehicles

A common source of partnership disagreements occurs over the way in which the ownership and running costs of motor cars are handled. There are often differing views between the senior and the junior partners on the number, value, type and size of cars that should be purchased or leased and the amount of private motoring that is undertaken by the individual partners and their spouses.

If cars are to be owned by individual partners it is their responsibility to maintain the vehicle in good running order. If one partner wishes to decide to own and maintain a more expensive motor car or drive a higher private mileage than the other partners, then an equitable method of adjustment or compensation between the partners should be agreed.

These motoring arrangements should be discussed and agreed in advance and a decision made as to whether the cars will be owned by the partnership or by each individual partner with the reimbursement of motoring costs by either payment of actual motor expenses or by means of a motoring allowance for business miles.

Loss of a driving licence can be very serious for veterinary surgeons in general practice who have to provide the public with a 24-hour service. It can be very expensive to have to hire a driver for a daily round of equine or large animal visits and in addition to provide rota cover for night and weekend work. It has now become commonplace to include a clause in the partnership agreement to the effect that if a partner is disqualified from driving a motor car, for any reason, including the totting up procedure, then that partner shall be personally responsibile for the paying of any fines and additional costs in arranging transport so that he or she can continue their normal practice duties.

Name of partnership

It used to be the custom to include all the partners' names in the practice title with each new partner having his name added on at the end of the list of names. This became impractical in larger practices and it also required regular changes in printed stationery.

Most practices now adopt a practice title that the public can identify with, such as the 'Abbeyfield Veterinary Group', 'Oaktree Animal Clinic' or 'Beaufort Equine Centre' and this title can continue irrespective of partnership changes. In choosing such a name care should be taken to select a title that will avoid confusion with other local veterinary practices in the area and not to give a misleading impression of the services provided.

However, the individual principal's or partners true names must be shown on all practice letterheads and invoices and displayed prominently at any premises where their business is carried on, and to which customers or suppliers have access.

The only professional premises that may be described as a veterinary hospital are those veterinary premises that have passed an inspection and have met the criteria and standards laid down by the Royal College and the British Veterinary Hospitals Association.

The title of specialist clinic may refer to an RCVS listed specialist only if a recognised RCVS specialist in that particular discipline is in charge of the service and provides it in person during advertised hours.

Part time working

With the greater influx of female graduates into the profession, more consideration should be given to the introduction of part time working and job sharing for all the partners. More senior partners may well consider working in the practice on a part time basis rather than taking early retirement.

Pensions

Most partnerships state that each partner shall be responsible for their own personal pension arrangements.

Residence occupation

Veterinary surgeons in practice have to maintain a 24-hour emergency service for the treatment of their clients' animals. It is therefore not unreasonable to ask that each partner lives close enough to the main premises or branch surgery so that he or she can provide a prompt service when on duty.

The actual distance will be decided on the time that it takes to travel in the practice area: which will vary between urban and rural districts, the time of day or night and the type of species that the practice deals with i.e. small animal, equine or farm.

Retirement

It is advantageous for both the senior and the junior partners that there should be a normal retirement age written into the agreement. A planned age for retirement allows the younger partners to make proper provision for the succession of the senior partner. It may be mutually advantageous for the senior partner to continue to work in the practice as a consultant on a part time basis after he has reached retirement age, subject to the consent of the other partners.

It is recommended that a clause should be included to avoid two partners or more seeking voluntary retirement together. When two partners wish to retire at the same time then a clause should stipulate a method to determine priority between the partners.

Revision of terms

It is advisable to agree that the terms of the partnership will be reviewed on a regular basis – say every three years. This will allow the partnership agreement to be discussed and updated between all the partners and is of particular importance with reference to covenants, cross insurance, termination, and the clauses relating to the valuation of property and goodwill.

Any changes from the original agreement will need to be agreed by unanimous decision and signed by all partners.

Termination of partnership

The circumstances under which a termination of the partnership may occur should be set out i.e. expulsion, illness, death or retirement. The details for the evaluation and payment of the practice assets by the remaining partners may vary according to the circumstances of the retirement.

A voluntary early retirement would be treated less favourably than a retirement from illness or by the death of a partner, where funds are more readily available from critical illness or cross insurance life policies. In some circumstances of termination, where all partners wish to retire then a dissolution may require that the practice is sold on the open market. Some practices will penalise early voluntary retirement by a reduction of the goodwill value or by extended repayment terms.

The *double option wording* is used as a device to reduce the risk that the estate of the deceased partner may be treated by the Inland Revenue as a mandatory purchase on death as being the equivalent to a cash payment which would not be eligible for inheritance tax relief; rather than a business asset, which is eligible for inheritance tax.

The valuation of the property is a constant source of difficulty between partners due to the wide variation of values obtained from estate agents and chartered surveyors. It is helpful to write into the partnership agreement the method of valuation that is to be used by a surveyor i.e. 'open market' value, 'on going' veterinary use or 'full development' value.

The valuation of goodwill can be the cause of dispute and problems can arise when a formula is used that becomes outdated. It is therefore advised that any stated method of goodwill valuation should be updated on a regular basis or the clause should state that the goodwill should be valued by an experienced valuer at current market price.

Index

accident book, 207
account clients, 163
accountants, 1, 121, 137
accounts, 121
   balance sheet, 125, 130
   fixed assets, 124
   invoice production, 145
   management, 112, 151
   partnership, 226
   payment of accounts, 146
   payment on time, 146
   profit and loss, 122, 123, 128
   source and application, 127, 132
   schedule of fixed assets, 129
   submission of accounts, 145, 164
advertising, 4, 90
amortisation, 139
animal charities, 25
annuity, 70
Ansoff's matrix, 92
anti-virus software, 109
appointments, 8, 73
   list, 111
appraisals, staff, 50, 52, 53, 54
arbitration, 238
architect, 1
assistants agreement, 4
assumptions, budgetting, 156, 163
audit of accounts, 121

back-up, 109
bad debt, 75
balance sheet, 125, 130
bank charges, 129, 144
   manager, 1
benefits in kind, 174
Blue Cross, 5
bonus schemes, 48
book debt, 62, 130
bookeeping records, 98
booster reminders, 8, 74, 113
Boston, matrix, 91
British Telecom, 5
BSAVA, 6, 19, 21, 48, 243
budget forecasts, 75, 134

   preparation, 134
   timetable, 135
business plan, 116
   marketing, 87
   records, 98
buying a partnership, 219
buying a property, 166
BVA, 4, 116, 207, 238, 239, 240
   animal welfare fund, 15, 21
   divisions, 6
   postgraduate symposium, 73
   slide kit, 24
   /SPVS annual survey, 117, 133, 136, 137
BVHA, 246

capital allowances, 132, 139
   budgeting, 138
   expenditure, 138, 140
   gains tax, 67, 68
   investment, 227
   investment analysis, 141
   payback period, 141
   payments, 227
   working, 132
carcase disposal, 5, 43, 204
caring attitude, 46
car parking, 7, 12
case history, 40
cash flow, 62, 135, 143
   discounted, 142
   forecasting, 135, 147
Cats Protection League, 5
CD ROM, 109, 115
chartered surveyor, 1, 169
CHIP Regulations, 202
client meetings, 19
   service, 9
clinical areas, 16
   examination, 8, 40
   records, 7, 40, 111
   waste, 203
communication, 93
companies, 201
   corporation tax, 217

open day, 25
  market option, 70
  market value, 67
  new surgery, 25

P's – four, 89
Pareto's Law, 88
partners, capital accounts, 126, 131
  finance, 62
  meetings, 75
  motor vehicles, 63
  personnel, 60
  practice promotion, 64
  responsibilities, 60
  rotas, 64
  salaried, 237
  stock, 221
partnership, accounts, 226
  buying-in, 219
  creditors, 223
  debtors, 223
  equipment, 220
  property, 220
  selling, 219
Partnership Act, 237
partnership, agreement, 237
  accident or sickness, 244
  arbitration, 238
  assets, 238
  binding out, 239
  business names, 237
  capital, 238
  cessation, 176
  contracts, 237
  covenants, 239
  decision making, 240
  dissolution, 241
  double option, 248
  drawings, 241
  driving disqualification, 242
  duration, 242
  duties, 241
  expulsion, 242
  firm name, 245
  goodwill, 222, 243
  guide, 239
  holidays, 243
  illness or incapacity, 244
  legacy, 245
  map of practice area, 239
  mediator, 238
  meetings, 78, 239

motor vehicles, 222, 245
  name, 245
  off duty, 243
  partners duties, 237, 241
  part time working, 246
  pension, 246
  pregnancy, 84, 207, 244
  profits, 239, 241
  residence occupation, 246
  restraint of practice, 239
  retirement, 66, 224, 247
  revision, 247
  spouses, 242
  succesion date, 247
  termination, 247
payback period, 141
PAYE, 3, 182
  codes, 182
  deduction sheet, 185
  end of year returns, 185
  P11D, 183
  P45, 183
PEP's, 168
pet health, phone-ins, 10
pet insurance, 2, 25, 35
petty cash, 143
PDSA, 5, 23
pensions, 190
  annuity, 70, 191
  AVC's, 192
  company, 192
  final salary, 192
  money purchase, 192
  open market option, 70, 191
  personal, 70, 173, 190
  SERPS, 190
  stakeholders, 173
  state, 69, 190
petcare, 18
  centre, 18
  counsellor, 18
  health, 18
  products, 18
petty cash, 143
pharmacy, 194
  cascade, 198
  containers, 196
  dispensing, 194
  labelling, 194, 196
  Medicines Act 1968, 194
PIW, 210
planning permission, 166

induction, 50
interviews, 57
job description, 74, 82
manual, 50
meetings, 9, 47
motivation, 45
name badges, 46
promotion, 46
sickness, absence, 84
teamwork, 47
training, 49
standard operating procedures, 61,
    103
start up practice, 1, 35, 134, 135, 175
State Incapacity Benefit, 69
stationery, 4
statutory sick pay, 210
stocks of drugs, 109
    control, 63, 102, 109
    current value, 128
    discounts, 104
    financial significance, 102
    forward buying, 104
    in hand, 147
    labelling, 196
    levels, 104, 131
    losses, 105
    ordering system, 102
    receipt procedure, 103
    stocktake, 130
    storage, 103
strategic planning, 88
surgery times, 13
survey, structural, 169
SWOT analysis, 117, 118

target marketing, 88
telephone, 26, 41
terms of trade, 164
time weighted average, 207
Town and Country Planning Act, 166
training, 50

transaction fee, 11
transfer of undertakings, 213

uniforms, 46, 86

valuation of property, 130, 169, 248
Value Added Tax, 3, 101, 150, 177
    annual accounting, 178
    annual threshold, 3, 177
    bad debt relief, 180
    car fuel scale, 179
    cash accounting, 179
    export schemes, 181
    inputs, 177
    inspector, 180
    penalties, 180
    records, 101, 177
    registration, 177
    returns, 112, 178
    special schemes, 178
Veterinary Defence Society, 186
veterinary nurse, 28, 29
    clinics, 35
    name badges, 29
    uniforms, 46, 86
veterinary surgeons attitude, 39
    client relationship, 39
    telephone, 41
virus, computer, 109
VMD, 199
VPMA, 78
    certificate, 78

waiting room, 13
what if, 113, 137
wildlife, 25, 48
word processing, 109
work chargeable hours, 158
working time regulations, 215

year to date, 136
Yellow Pages, 5, 76